MULTIDISCIPLINARY APPROACH TO THE MANAGEMENT OF OBESITY

Handbook for Physicians and Health Care Professionals

MULTIDISCIPLINARY APPROACH TO THE MANAGEMENT OF

OBESITY

Handbook for Physicians and Health Care Professionals

Lalita Kaul, PhD, RD, LD, LN
Joseph J Nidiry, MD
Henry W Williams, Jr, MD, MPH

Howard University College of Medicine
Department of Community Health
and Family Practice
Washington, DC

Medical
and
Engineering
Publishers, Inc

First published in the United States of America by
Medical and Engineering Publishers, Inc
PO Box 74
Sunshine, MD 20833-0074
USA
(http://www.mepublishers.com)

Library of Congress Cataloging-in-Publication Data

Multidisciplinary Approach to the Management of Obesity
Handbook for Physicians and Health Care Professionals
Lalita Kaul, Joseph J Nidiry, Henry W Williams. First Edition
Includes bibliographical references and index
2005

Library of Congress Control Number: 2005924374
ISBN 978-1-930636-04-0

Printed in USA.

Printed on acid-free paper.

To my daughter, Kavita, whose continuous support and encouragement sustained me in completion of this book.

Lalita Kaul

ACKNOWLEDGEMENTS

My special thanks go to Ms. Ruth Matthews for her assistance in putting the book manuscript together. Technical and editorial assistance of Mrs. Sharon Whitt from Medical and Engineering Publishers, Inc. is also greatly acknowledged.

My life has been enriched over the years by my students, residents, colleagues, clients, and patients; their contributions are revealed in my work. Each one has taught me something about human experience, and I am grateful for those opportunities.

And finally, but most of all, I am grateful for the support of my husband, Dr. Dali J. Patel, who stimulated me enormously in this project.

Lalita Kaul

DISCLAIMER

Contents

Appendices

PREFACE

Nutrition is becoming a primary force in preventive medicine and clinical research has implicated nutritional factors in a number of the most prevalent diseases in the United States. Some of these include coronary heart disease, non-insulin dependent diabetes mellitus, cancer, arteriosclerosis, and alcohol induced cirrhosis. In addition, dietary habits are associated with prevention and treatment of diseases, including obesity, low birth weight, and osteoporosis.

Until recently, obesity was considered to be a rather benign condition not necessarily requiring treatment. This attitude has gradually been changing as the prevalence of the condition has increased remarkably and the health risks have been recognized. In the United States, the costs to the society of obesity have been estimated to be 68.8 billion dollars.

A sedentary lifestyle and the variety of tasty, rich, and cheap foods available in the United States make Americans particularly vulnerable to weight gain. It is now clear that obesity is to some extent biologically determined and that approximately 25% to 40% of the tendency toward obesity is caused by genetics. This leaves a great portion of the variance attributable to environment, and therefore, much can be done to improve this condition.

Persuading people to eat a healthier diet for obesity prevention or treatment is one of the greatest challenges to medical and public health care among providers. Each year physicians see 70 percent of all adults in the United States, who represent an immediately available resource for physicians to encourage health promotion and disease prevention. Yet there exist numerous incongruities between physicians' actions regarding dietary recommendations and the recommended guidelines, despite the population-wide potential for modifying dietary risk factors for various diseases.

Barriers to successful physician-delivered dietary counseling by physicians in both the US and Canada have included lack of training in nutrition, lack of time, lack of support staff with nutrition training, and reimbursement concerns. Additional factors include beliefs about the effectiveness of intervention, concerns about patient response and compliance, knowledge about risk factors and perceived unpalatableness of certain diets. Survey data have revealed that physicians who feel prepared and competent to offer dietary counseling are more likely to be willing to intervene around dietary practices to provide dietary counseling to their patients. Although physicians are thought by many to be in an advantageous position to promote healthy lifestyle, few physicians place emphasis on diet. Medical educators have felt that improving the nutrition education of physicians would increase the inclusion of nutrition in patient care. However, having the knowledge does not necessarily guarantee appropriate nutrition related patient care.

Washington, DC

Lalita Kaul
Joseph J Nidiry
Henry W Williams, Jr

Chapter 1

INTRODUCTION

More than half of the US population is overweight (BMI >25 kg/m^2) or obese (BMI >30 kg/m^2), providing physicians, nurses and dietitians more an opportunity to work with this medical problem. Obesity is a chronic condition and should be treated as such. A standard model may not help every obese patient because there are often many complex issues (hereditary factors, the environment, and psychological factors) that differ between patients [1, 24, 30, 70].

Successful treatment of obesity seldom requires that the individual return to their "*ideal*" body weight. Permanent loss of as little as 5% body weight can result in substantial, long-term improvements in health. Therefore, the focus of obesity treatment should be on the permanent maintenance of a realistic lower body weight rather than a rapid weight loss to ideal level.

Most of the physicians have much of the information needed to assess whether weight management intervention is warranted.

APPROACH TO THE OVERWEIGHT/OBESE PATIENT

Baseline information – examination/office records

Height and weight – this is a means for rapidly assessing the patient's potential need for intervention. The first step is to have the patient's Body Mass Index (BMI).

Although seldom measured in an office setting, the waist circumference is a reasonable indicator of abdominal (high-risk) fat, and will further help characterize the patient's health risk from obesity. The presence of obesity or overweight with a waist circumference >102 cm (40 inches) in men or 88 cm (35 inches) in women suggests the need for treatment, especially in the presence of obesity-related health problems.

Blood pressure measurement may be a routine part of an office visit, but if not taken with an appropriate (large) cuff, the reading may be falsely elevated. Given the prevalence of obesity, it is not unreasonable to have large blood pressure cuffs available in most health care settings.

The availability of these routine measures should assist the health care providers in determining whether or not to discuss the issue of overweight or obesity with their patient.

Discussing the Problem – making it easier for the patient

Physicians who are familiar with obesity evaluation and treatment may perceive that there is little time to intervene during a brief office visit. Another concern is that mentioning the patient's weight may cause the patient to withdraw or respond negatively. Physicians are uniquely positioned, however, to provide weight and nutrition intervention. Patients who receive effective messages from their physicians are more likely to follow through on recommended changes in lifestyle. For example, in less than one minute the physician can point out that lifestyle changes (improved eating habits, increased physical activity) can help in the management of diabetes, hypertension or lipid disorders. The smoking cessation model is a good example of how focused and clear messages given by physicians to patients repeatedly over time can result in significant benefits with modest efforts. If the patient is receptive, a referral can quickly be made to a dietitian or other health professional with expertise in weight management.

If a physician is to be effective in intervening to help the obese patients, he/she must be sensitive to the communication issues with these patients. Creating a supportive medical environment for the obese patients can make communication easier. For example, having available larger examining gowns, weighing scales, blood pressure cuffs, and examining tables may be appropriate if the physician sees a significant number of obese patients.

The physician's office staff may need to be educated regarding sensitivity and privacy issues. These issues include location of the scale and references to a patient's weight by the staff. Both the office staff and the physician need to have empathy for the obese patient and to communicate with the patient in an unbiased and supportive manner.

Medical History Relevant to Obesity

Medical conditions that are affected by obesity (diabetes, dyslipidemia, hypertension, sleep apnea, etc) can be a good starting point for discussion of weight-related issues. Documenting blood pressure, blood lipid and glucose concentrations should be standard data collection for obesity management. Degenerative joint disease is clearly aggravated by being overweight and should be noted. Perhaps the most commonly overlooked complication of obesity is obstructive sleep apnea. Patients should be asked about excessive daytime sleepiness and related symptoms. Spouses often can provide important clues regarding the diagnosis of sleep apnea. Referral to a sleep disorder specialist can be extremely helpful, as the treatments for sleep apnea are remarkably effective.

Medications predisposing to weight gain (steroids, antidepressants, thiazolidinediones, some antihistamines and anticonvulsants) should be assessed because beginning weight management programs may be fruitless depending upon the medication.

A family history of obesity and obesity-related medical problems can assist in prognosticating obesity-related health complications.

A brief consideration that secondary causes of obesity (Cushing's syndrome, psychiatric disturbances) may be present is usually warranted. Excluding secondary causes of obesity is generally a straightforward process that can be addressed by a directed history and physical examination. A long duration of overweight and positive family history of obesity makes it unlikely that a secondary cause exists. Exogenous corticosteroids and tricyclic antidepressants are the more common medications resulting in unwanted weight gain, and weight loss is more difficult if these medications are continued. Physical signs that would indicate a secondary cause of obesity, such as Cushing's syndrome, should be sought. The absence of a positive family history of obesity is unusual and should prompt a more thorough search for secondary causes, including emotional disturbances.

Even if there are medical indications for obesity treatment, it is important to assess whether the patients are ready to change their lifestyle in attempts to deal with the issue. Only if they are willing to try is a further effort on the health care provider's part likely to be helpful.

If the patient is willing to work with treatment, a review of the patient's goals and expectations are warranted. Unrealistic goals can lead to disappointment for all involved. Additional information that can help in developing a program include the pattern of weight gain, including inciting events, the response to previous weight loss attempts, as well as the patient's eating pattern and activity habits.

Physical examination

The physical examination is largely directed towards searching for clues of secondary causes of weight gain (physical stigmata of Cushing's syndrome or hypothyroidism) and documenting complications of obesity or obesity-related diseases. A careful examination of the skin and cardiovascular system is most likely to yield clues to the patient's condition.

Laboratory evaluation/tests

In routine clinical practice, assessment of blood glucose (diabetes), cholesterol, triglycerides and HDL-cholesterol (dyslipidemia), and liver function tests (steatohepatitis) will provide the needed information to assess the most common health-related issues.

Chapter 2

PREVALENCE OF OBESITY

The United States is experiencing substantial increases in overweight and obesity (as defined by a BMI ≥ 25 for adults) that cut across all ages, racial and ethnic groups, and both genders. According to self-reported measures of height and weight, obesity (BMI ≥ 30) has been increasing in every State in the Nation. Based on clinical height and weight measurements in the 1999 National Health and Nutrition Examination Survey (NHANES), 34 percent of US adults aged 20 to 74 years are overweight (BMI 25 to 29.9), and an additional 27 percent are obese (BMI ≥ 30) [4, 5, 7-12, 14, 37, 95]. This contrasts with the late 1970s, when an estimated 32 percent of adults aged 20 to 74 years were overweight, and 15 percent were obese (Figure 1).

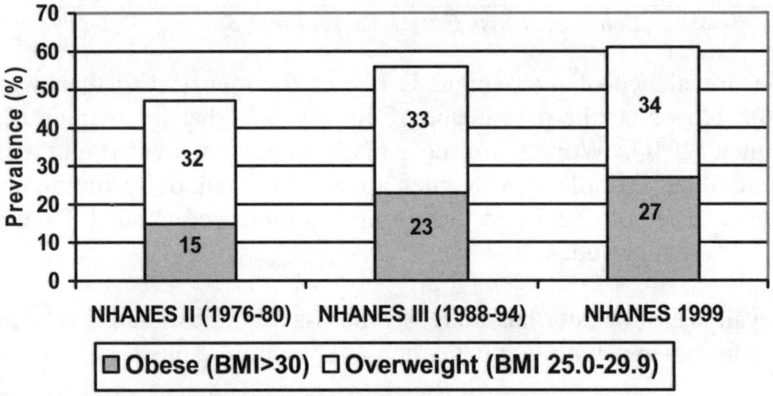

FIGURE 1

Age adjusted prevalence of overweight and obesity among US adults aged 20 to 74 years

Source: *Centers for Disease Control and Prevention (CDC), National Center for Health Statistics (NCHS), National Health and Nutrition Examination Survey (NHANES)*

According to NHANES III Survey, 10-15% of children and adolescents are overweight. This change in the prevalence of overweight can be accounted for only by environmental factors. There is alteration in the balance of dietary intake and physical activity levels of children and adolescents. This rapid increase in the prevalence of overweight in children and adolescents has shown an increase in obesity-associated chronic diseases. About 60% of overweight children from 5 to 10 years have hypelipidemia, elevated blood pressure or hyperinsulinemia. Those children will require effective treatment to prevent obesity in adulthood (Table 1).

TABLE 1
Obesity Prevalence (1991 and 1998)

Age (Years)	1991 Obesity Prevalence (%)	1998 Obesity Prevalence (%)
18-29	7.1	12.1
30-39	11.3	16.9
40-49	15.8	21.2
50-59	16.1	23.8
60-69	14.7	21.3
≥ 70	11.4	14.6

Source: *Behavioral Risk Factor Surveillance System, 1991-1998*

The prevalence of overweight is higher for men (59%) than women (51%). However, the prevalence of obesity is higher for women (25%) than men (20%). Women are more likely to become overweight as they become older. Middle-aged women are at a high risk of becoming obese. The prevalence of obesity in this group has increased about 1% per year over a 34-year period.

Prevalence of obesity has increased across all educational levels and is higher for persons with less education as shown in Table 2.

TABLE 2
Obesity Prevalence and Educational Levels

Education Level	1991 Obesity Prevalence (%)	1998 Obesity Prevalence (%)
< High School	16.5	24.1
High School	13.3	19.4
Some College	10.6	17.8
College	8.0	13.1

Source: *Behavioral Risk Factor Surveillance System, 1991-1998*

Obesity prevalence has increased across all US regions as shown in Table 3.

TABLE 3
Percentage of Adults with Obesity in the US by Region

Region of the US*	1991 (%)	1998 (%)
New England (Connecticut, Massachusetts, Maine, New Hampshire, Vermont)	9.9	14.4
Middle Atlantic (New Jersey, New York, Pennsylvania)	12.7	16.7
East North Central (Illinois, Indiana, Michigan, Ohio, Wisconsin)	14.1	19.1
West North Central (Iowa, Minnesota, Missouri, North Dakota, Nebraska, South Dakota)	12.2	18.0
South Atlantic (Delaware, Florida, Georgia, Maryland, North Carolina, South Carolina, Virginia, West Virginia)	11.1	18.6
East South Central (Alabama, Kentucky, Mississippi, Tennessee)	13.1	20.0
West South Central (Louisiana, Oklahoma, Texas)	13.1	19.9
Mountain (Arizona, Colorado, Idaho, Montana, New Mexico, Utah)	9.6	14.1
Pacific (Alaska, California, Hawaii, Oregon, Washington)	10.2	17.0

Source: *Behavioral Risk Factor Surveillance System, 1991-1998*
**Arkansas, District of Columbia, Kansas, Nevada, Rhode Island, and Wyoming are excluded since weight and height were not collected for one or more years.*

DISPARITIES IN PREVALENCE

Overweight and obesity in the US occur at higher rates in African Americans and Hispanic Americans, compared with White Americans. Asian Americans have relatively low prevalence for obesity. Women and persons of low socioeconomic status appear to particularly be affected by overweight and obesity.

PREVALENCE

- The prevalence of overweight [Body Mass Index (BMI) of 25 or more] increased over the last decade across racial/ethnic groups as shown in Table 4.
- Mexican American and African American (non-Hispanic) adults in the US are considerably overweight and obese than white (non-Hispanic) adults.
- The American Indian population also has high prevalence rates of overweight and obesity. Rates for American Indians in Arizona were at 80 percent for women and 67 percent for men.

TABLE 4
Increase in Overweight and Obesity Prevalence Among US Adults* by Racial/Ethnic Group

	Overweight (BMI ≥ 25) Prevalence (%)		Obesity (BMI ≥ 30) Prevalence (%)	
Racial/Ethnic Group	1988 to 1994	1999 to 2000	1988 to 1994	1999 to 2000
African American (non-Hispanic)	62.5	69.6	30.2	39.9
Mexican American	67.4	73.4	28.4	34.4
White (non-Hispanic)	52.6	62.3	21.2	28.7

Source: *CDC, National Center for Health Statistics, National Health and Nutrition Examination Survey. Flegal, et al. JAMA 2002: 288: 1723-1727 and IJO 1998:22:39-47*

**Ages 20 and older for 1999 to 2000 and ages 20 to 74 for 1988 to 1994*

GENDER

- For women, the African American (non-Hispanic) population has the highest prevalence of overweight and obesity.

- For men, the Mexican American population has the highest prevalence of overweight and obesity as shown in Tables 5 and 6.
- Overweight, obesity and severe obesity (BMI of 40 or more) prevalence increased in women in various racial/ethnic groups in the US over the last decade as shown in Table 7.

TABLE 5
Increase in Overweight (BMI ≥ 25) Prevalence among US Adults (Ages 20 to 74) by Racial/Ethnic Group and Gender

	Men Prevalence (%)		Women Prevalence (%)	
Racial/Ethnic Group	1988 to 1994	1999 to 2000	1988 to 1994	1999 to 2000
African American (non-Hispanic)	58.2	60.1	68.5	78
Mexican American	69.4	74.4	69.6	71.8
White (non-Hispanic)	61.6	67.5	47.2	57.5

Source: *CDC, National Center for Health Statistics, National Health and Nutrition Examination Survey. Health, United States (Table 70) 2002*

TABLE 6
Increase in Obesity (BMI ≥ 30) Prevalence among US Adults (Ages 20 to 74) by Racial/Ethnic Group and Gender

	Men Prevalence (%)		Women Prevalence (%)	
Racial/Ethnic Group	1988 to 1994	1999 to 2000	1988 to 1994	1999 to 2000
African American (non-Hispanic)	21.3	28.8	39.1	50.8
Mexican American	24.4	29.4	36.1	40.1
White (non-Hispanic)	20.7	27.7	23.3	30.6

Source: *CDC, National Center for Health Statistics, National Health and Nutrition Examination Survey. Health, United States (Table 70) 2002*

TABLE 7
Increase in Severe Obesity (BMI ≥ 40) Prevalence among US Adults (Ages 20 and older) by Racial/Ethnic Group and Gender

	Overweight (BMI ≥ 25) Prevalence (%)		Obesity (BMI ≥ 30) Prevalence (%)	
Racial/Ethnic Group	1988 to 1994	1999 to 2000	1988 to 1994	1999 to 2000
African American (non-Hispanic)	2.4	3.5	7.9	15.1
Mexican American	1.1	2.4	4.8	5.5
White (non-Hispanic)	1.8	3	3.4	4.9

Source: *CDC, National Center for Health Statistics, National Health and Nutrition Examination Survey. Flegal, et al. JAMA. 2002:288:1723-172*

SOCIOECONOMIC STATUS

- Overweight affects African American women and men across all SES levels.
- Minority women with low income appear to have the greatest likelihood of being obese.
- Among Mexican American women, age 20 to 74, the rate of overweight is higher for women living below the poverty line versus above the poverty line.

HEALTH DISPARITIES

Many obesity-related diseases included diabetes, hypertension, cancer and heart disease are found in higher rates among various members of racial-ethnic minorities compared to whites [97, 98].

Diabetes

- Diabetes has been reported to occur at a rate of 16 to 26 percent in Hispanic and African Americans, aged 45 to 74, compared with 12 percent in white of the same age.
- Higher BMI predicts the risk for type 2 diabetes in Pima Indians.
- Among 15 American Indian tribes studied in Oklahoma, 77 percent of adults with diabetes are reported to be obese.

- Among Mexican Americans, obesity and type 2 diabetes are both increasing risk factor of cardiovascular disease including smoking and blood pressure.

Heart Disease

- Among African Americans, the high prevalence of obesity and obesity-related disease such as hypertension and type 2 diabetes, are factors reported to contributed to death rate from coronary heart disease.
- In a study of older Hispanics, with an average age of 80, obesity was found to be a factor for developing coronary artery disease.

Hypertension

- The high prevalence of obesity is reported to be a contributing factor to the prevalence of hypertension in minority populations, especially among African Americans who have an earlier onset and run a more severe course of hypertension.

Behavioral Risk Factors Diet and Exercise

- Cultural factors related to dietary choices, physical activity, and acceptance weight among African Americans and other racial-ethnic groups, appear to be interfering with weight loss efforts.
- Sedentary life style, which can contribute to the development of obesity, has been reported by 44 to 60 percent of Native American men.

One in four adults below the poverty level is obese, compared with 1 in 6 in households with an income of $67,000 or more. The assumption use to be that the poor were making bad food and lifestyle choices – doughnuts instead of whole wheat bread. Cheap foods tend to be based with sugar, fat and refined grains (cookies and chocolate bars). In general, processed foods are larger portions of all American diets. A pound of lean steak costs lots more than a pound of hot dogs. Processed foods are cheap, tasty, filling and more accessible. Poor people wind up buying much of their daily groceries from convenience stores. Some communities are trying to remedy this by opening more supermarkets in urban neighborhoods.

Chapter 3

CHILDHOOD AND ADOLESCENT OBESITY

The most recent 1999 data estimate that 13 percent of children aged 6 to 11 years and 14 percent of adolescents aged 12 to 19 years are overweight. [66, 156, 157]. During the past two decades, the percentage of children who are overweight has nearly doubled (from 7 to 13 percent), and the percentage of adolescents who are overweight has almost tripled (from 5 to 14 percent) (Figure 1).

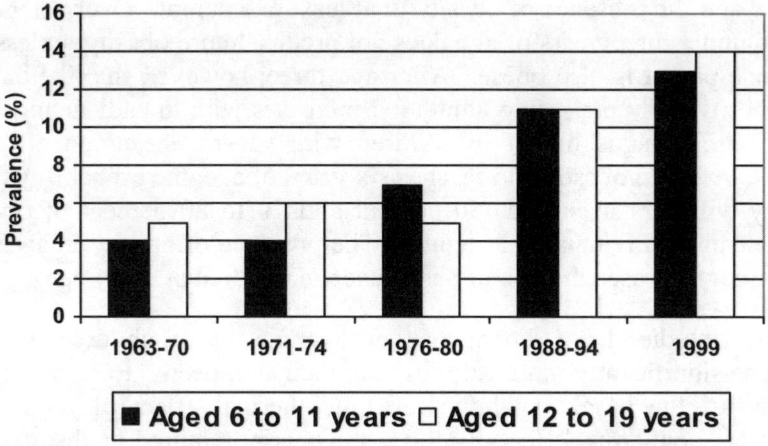

FIGURE 1

Prevalence of Overweight* among US Children and Adolescents
**Gender- and age-specific BMI≥ the 95th percentile*
Source: *Centers for Disease Control and Prevention (CDC), National Center for Health Statistics (NCHS) National Health Examination Survey (NHES), National Health and Nutrition Examination Survey (NHANES)*

In many obese people, the roots of their disorder can be traced back to childhood. Obesity tends to continue throughout life, its presence at any age will increase the risk of persistence at subsequent ages. While most obese infants will not remain so, they are at increased risk of becoming obese children. These children are in turn more likely to become obese adolescents, who are then very likely to remain obese as adults.

Evaluation of obesity in childhood is important for several reasons. First, it offers the best hope for preventing disease progression with its associated morbidities into adulthood. Second, while genetic and hormonal causes of obesity are rare, they do warrant consideration in obese children. In addition, obesity has a negative impact on the self-esteem of children and adolescents. Emphasizing healthy eating and exercise habits for children and their families may have lasting effects on the lifestyle of these patients.

The persistence of obesity into adulthood depends on several factors, including the age at which the child becomes obese, the severity of the disease and the presence of obesity in at least one parent. Overweight in a child under three years of age does not predict future obesity, unless at least one parent is also obese. After age three, however, the likelihood that obesity will persist into adulthood increases with the advancing age of the child and is higher in children with severe obesity in all age groups. After an obese child reaches six years of age, the probability that obesity will persist exceeds 50 percent and 70 to 80 percent of obese adolescents will remain so as adults. The presence of obesity in at least one parent increases the risk of persistence in children at every age.

Several studies have shown that, on average, obese children do not consume significantly more calories than their thin peers. Energy output consists of the basal metabolic rate, the thermal effect of food and activity. The thermal effect of food is the energy required to absorb and digest meals. Activity is the least influenced by genetic inheritance and is therefore the one most susceptible to change. About 3500 Calories is equivalent to 1 lb; thus, an excess intake of only 50 to 100 Calories per day will lead to a five- to 10-lb weight gain over one year. As a result, a relatively small imbalance between energy input and output can lead to significant weight gain over time. Most obese children demonstrate a slow but consistent weight gain over several years.

EVALUATION OF OBESE CHILDREN AND ADOLESCENTS

Only a small percentage of childhood obesity is associated with a hormonal or genetic defect, with the remainder being idiopathic in nature. The most common of the endogenous causes of childhood obesity and their associated characteristics are listed in Table 1. An endogenous cause for obesity can be either suspected or eliminated from the differential diagnosis in virtually all children based on a careful history and physical examination. In most cases, this should negate the need for expensive and unnecessary laboratory evaluations. Genetic syndromes are listed in Table 2.

TABLE 1
Endogenous Causes of Childhood and Adolescent Obesity

Hormonal causes	**Diagnostic clues**
Hypothyroidism	(Increased TSH, decreased thyroxin T_4) levels
Hypercortisolism	Abnormal dexamethasone suppression test; increased 24-hour free urinary cortisol level
Primary hyperinsulinism	Increased plasma insulin, increased C-peptide levels
Pseudohypoparathyroidism	Hypocalcemia, hyperphosphatemia, increased PTH level
Acquired hypothalamic	Presence of hypothalamic tumor, infection, syndrome trauma, vascular lesion

TABLE 2
Genetic Syndromes Associated with Childhood and Adolescent Obesity

Genetic syndromes	**Associated characteristics**
Prader-Willi	Obesity, unsatiable appetite, mental retardation, hypogonadism, strabismus
Laurence-Moon/Bardet-Biedl	Obesity, mental retardation, pigmentary retinopathy, hypogonadism, spastic paraplegia

Alstrom	Obesity, retinitis pigmentosa, deafness, diabetes mellitus
Borjeson-Forssman-Lehmann	Obesity, mental retardation, hypogonadism, hypometabolism, epilepsy
Cohen	Truncal obesity, mental retardation, hypotonia
Turner's	Short stature, undifferentiated gonads, cardiac abnormalities, webbed neck, obesity, 45, X genotype
Familial Lipodystrophy	Muscular hypertrophy, acromegalic appearance, liver enlargement, acanthosis nigricans, insulin resistance, hypertriglyceridemia, mental retardation
Beckwith-Wiedemann	Gigantism, exomphalos, macroglossia, visceromegaly
Sotos'	Cerebral gigantism, physical overgrowth, hypotonia, delayed motor and cognitive development
Weaver	Infant overgrowth syndrome, accelerated skeletal maturation, unusual facies
Ruvalcaba	Mental retardation, microcephaly, skeletal abnormalities, hypogonadism, brachymetapody
Gene associations	
Leptin	
$Beta_3$-adrenergic receptor	
TSH=*Thyroid-stimulating hormone*; **PTH**=*parathyroid hormone*	

Growth failure characterizes endogenous obesity. Children with an associated genetic or hormonal syndrome are short, usually at or under the 5th percentile of height for age. Children with idiopathic obesity are taller, usually above the 50th percentile. Even the onset of a hormonal abnormality in a previously tall child will be marked by a significantly slower rate of growth compared with the child's previous growth curve. Table 3 compares the important differences in the history and physical examination of patients with endogenous and idiopathic obesity.

TABLE 3
Characteristics of Idiopathic and Endogenous Obesity

Idiopathic obesity	Endogenous obesity
>90 percent of cases	<10 percent of cases
Tall stature (usually >50th percentile)	Short stature (usually <5th percentile)
Family history of obesity common	Family history of obesity uncommon
Mental function normal	Often mentally impaired
Normal or advanced bone age	Delayed bone age
Physical examination otherwise normal	Associated stigmata on physical examination

Although rarely encountered, hypothyroidism is the most frequently considered endogenous abnormality in obese children. By itself, hypothyroidism seldom causes massive weight gain, and its prevalence in obese patients does not significantly differ from is prevalence in the rest of the population. When present, hypothyroidism is usually associated with other signs and symptoms of the disease, such as constipation, cold intolerance, and dry skin. If this disorder is suspected, a thyroid-stimulating hormone (TSH) level should be determined.

Hypercortisolism (Cushing's syndrome) is another frequently suspected cause of endogenous obesity. Although it is usually iatrogenic in nature, it can also be secondary to adrenal tumors or primary pituitary overproduction of adrenocorticotropic hormone (ACTH). Pediatric hypercortisolism is characterized by linear growth failure and generalized weight gain. If this condition is suspected, the patient can be evaluated with a 24-hour urine cortisol collection or a dexamethasone-suppression test.

Office Evaluation

Obese children must be evaluated for associated morbidity. This includes an assessment of cardiac risk factors, weight-related orthopedic problems, skin disorders and potential psychiatric sequelae [151].

Cardiac risk factors include a family history of early cardiovascular disease, high cholesterol and blood pressure levels, cigarette smoking, the presence of diabetes mellitus, and decreased physical activity. Obesity in childhood is known to be associated with abnormal indices of lipolysis, including high cholesterol levels (greater than 170 mg per dl), high triglyceride levels and low levels of high-density lipoprotein. The National Cholesterol Education Program Expert Panel on Blood Cholesterol Levels in Children and Adolescents therefore recommends that physicians consider screening all obese children over two years of age for elevated cholesterol levels.

Obese children also have increased average blood pressure, heart rate, and cardiac output when compared to non-obese peers. When evaluating blood pressure in obese children, use of an appropriately sized blood pressure cuff is essential, because one that is too small may yield falsely elevated readings. Tobacco use should be ascertained in all adolescents, as this represents an independent risk for cardiovascular disease. Finally, the presence of diabetes should be considered in all morbidity obese children. While overt type 2 diabetes mellitus is rare in childhood, hyperinsulinemia and glucose intolerance are nearly universal in morbidly obese children.

The child's level of physical activity must also be assessed. This is important not only for cardiac risk evaluation but also to help guide future treatment. As a corollary to this, television viewing patterns should be reviewed, as television viewing has been shown to be associated with obesity in childhood.

Because they carry excess weight, obese children are at increased risk for orthopedic problems. These include tibial torsion and bowed legs, slipped capital femoral epiphysis (especially in boys) and symptoms of weight stress in the joints of the lower extremities.

Obese children are much more prone to skin disorders than are non-obese children, especially if deep skin folds are present. These disorders include heat rash, monilial dermatitis, and acanthosis nigricans (a condition that may be a marker for type 2 diabetes). In addition, acne should be treated when present, as this may help improve the child's self-image.

It is essential to address any existing psychiatric problems, including depression, poor self-esteem, negative self-image, and withdrawal from peers. From an early age, society stigmatizes obese children as lazy, stupid, slow, and self-indulgent. Studies have shown that children express negative attitude toward their obese peers as early as kindergarten, and that they prefer a playmate that is bound to a wheelchair or disabled by a major physical handicap to one who is obese. There is a clear association between obesity and low self-esteem, especially in adolescents. During the office visit, it is imperative that physicians be sensitive to and accepting of these patients, focusing on positive aspects and ensuring that treatment plans will not further damage an already fragile sense of self-esteem.

TREATMENT

The best way to significantly affect the prevalence of obesity is to prevent it. Therefore, the issue of obesity should be addressed during every well-child examination. Parents should know that both bottle- and breast-fed infants can be overfed, although overfeeding is more common in infants fed by bottle. Parents should be taught to respect their child's appetite and to understand that it is not necessary for an infant to finish every bottle. Breast feeding and delaying the introduction of solid foods may decrease the risk of future weight problems.

Skim milk can safely replace whole milk after two years of age. Food should not be used for non-nutritive purposes such as comfort or reward. Children should not be offered sweets as a reward for finishing a meal, as this teaches them to place a higher value on dessert foods and may make desserts more desirable to them. Family meals should be oriented toward a healthy diet with 30 percent or less of calories derived from fat. Finally, parents should limit the amount of television that the child is allowed to watch and should encourage active play in its place.

Weight loss goals should be realistic and should allow for normal growth. Goals should initially be small, so that the child doesn't become overwhelmed or discouraged. Five to 10 lbs is a reasonable first goal or, if preferred, a rate of 1 to 4 pounds per month can be established [88, 129].

DIETARY MANAGEMENT

The child should maintain a food record to aid in dietary assessment. The food diary should include not only the type and quantity of food eaten, but also where it was eaten, the time of day, and who else was present. In most cases, the diary will be inaccurate in figuring total Calories consumed but will be useful in reviewing problem foods and eating patterns. A straightforward dietary prescription should be offered, keeping in mind that 3500 Calories must be eliminated by diet and exercise to lose one pound. It is necessary to provide parents with a specific Calorie-per-day recommendation that follows guidelines for percentages of fat, protein, and carbohydrates. Dietary fiber is also important, as it increases satiety and displaces fat in the diet. The patient and family should be referred to books that describe the nutritional contents of foods and food exchange lists such as Exchange Lists for Weight Management. Finally, the patient and his family should be referred to a nutritional consultant, if this service is available in the community.

EXERCISE

Exercise is necessary to maintain weight loss and to redistribute body fat into muscle. It is, therefore, an essential part of any weight management program. Initial exercise recommendations should be small and exercise levels should be increased slowly, to avoid possible discouragement. A reasonable goal is 20 to 30 minutes of moderate activity per day, in addition to whatever exercise the child gets during the school day.

BEHAVIOR MODIFICATION

Self-monitoring is accomplished by food and activity logs, which force to become more aware of his or her eating and exercise patterns. Nutritional education should be aimed at both the child and the family. It should include the components of a healthy diet and an understanding of food labels and the importance of dietary fiber. The patient should be taught that 3500 Calories equals one lb; there are nine calories per gram of fat and only four calories per gram of carbohydrate or protein. Furthermore, 25 percent of the energy from carbohydrates will be used in its conversion and storage as fat in the body.

Stimulus control includes limiting the amount of fattening foods in the house, eating all meals at the dinner table and at designated times, and serving food only once before putting it away (no second helpings). Parents should not verbally encourage the child to eat, and the child should not be forced to finish the entire meal. Examples of modifying eating behavior include taking smaller bites, chewing food longer, putting the fork down between bites, and leaving some food on the plate.

Activity patterns are an important target for behavior modification. The child should help set a weekly activity goal, sign a contract to perform the activity, and help determine the reward for reaching the goal. Family television-viewing patterns should be reviewed and modified accordingly. Attitude change involves teaching the child to turn negative self-statements into positive ones, and helping him or her cope with the negative remarks of others. Finally, reinforcements and rewards include verbal praise from the physician and family members, as well as tangible rewards for achieving dietary, activity and weight-loss goals. Rewards should be determined with input from the child, and they should encourage further physical activity, such as sporting equipment or a trip to the skating rink.

FAMILY INVOLVEMENT

It is important to involve the entire family when treating obesity in children. Many studies have demonstrated a familial aggregation of risk factors for obesity, and the family provides the child's major social learning environment. It has been demonstrated that the long-term (10-year) effectiveness of a weight control program is significantly improved when the intervention is directed at the parents as well as the child, rather than aimed at the child alone.

ALTERNATIVE THERAPIES

At this time no anorexiant medications are approved by the US Food and Drug Administration for use in children. Surgical procedures such as gastric bypass have not been studied sufficiently in children to advise their use. Structured weight loss programs such as Weight Watchers and Jenny Craig Weight Loss Centers will accept older children with permission from their parents and physician. The components of a successful weight loss plan are given in Table 4.

TABLE 4
Components of a Successful Weight Loss Plan

1.	Reasonable weight loss goal
2.	Being in treatment as early as possible, preferably before adolescence
3.	Health professionals should educate families about the medical complications of obesity
4.	All family and significant caregivers should be involved in the treatment program
5.	Treatment programs should promote long-term permanent changes instead of short-term diets or exercise programs aimed at rapid weight loss
6.	The treatment program should include activities that help families learn to monitor eating and physical activity behavior.
7.	The treatment program should emphasize small, gradual changes. For example, the practitioner should recommend two or three specific changes in diet or activity at a time
8.	Health professionals should provide encouragement, rather than criticism and penalties
9.	A variety of health professionals should be involved in the weight management program. Physicians, nurses, nurse practitioners, dietetics professionals, social workers, and exercise physiologist can work together to effectively help families monitor and change behavior
10.	Group meetings may be efficient and effective

If a child fails to lose weight despite what appears to be adequate treatment, it is important to refrain from accusing the child of cheating on the diet or misreporting physical activity. Rather, a way out of the weight loss program should be offered. Many of these children have already experienced several perceived failures in their lives, and an unsuccessful attempt to lose weight should not be added to their emotional burden. They should be seen by a therapist.

Chapter 4

CAUSES OF OBESITY

BIOLOGY OF WEIGHT REGULATION

Body weight is regulated with caloric intake and energy expenditure. Obesity results from the failure of this regulatory system, with an imbalance between total energy intake and expenditure. It is induced by some combination of genetic, environmental and psychological influences. Regulation of body weight appears to be coordinated primarily by the hypothalamus, which receives afferent information from several sources. Circulating levels of the adipocyte-derived hormone, leptin, signal body energy stores. Through neurohumoral mechanism, the gastrointestinal tract provides information about recent food ingestion, and the cerebral cortex contributes behavioral information and regulation. Most people appear to maintain their weight around a physiological set point, and it is thought that obesity results in part from a disturbance in this control system (the mechanism of which is not known). Significant deviation from the set point leads to appropriate compensatory responses – weight loss causes a simultaneous drive for energy conservation (decreased expenditure) and increased caloric intake (increased hunger). Forced overeating generates the opposite effects [19, 83].

The effector arms of hypothalamic control of body weight include the regulation of food intake, metabolic activity, and energy expenditure (primarily in muscle and fat tissues). Among the many mediators of these regulatory systems are neuropeptide Y, insulin, and the sympathetic nervous system.

It is likely that obesity represents the manifestations of a spectrum of different disorders, each arising from distinct defects (or groups of defects) in the cortical (including psychological), hypothalamic, endocrine and/or metabolic components of the weight regulatory system.

DEFINITION OF OBESITY

Obesity is defined as an excess accumulation of fat in the body. In normal adults, fat constitutes 15 to 22% of the body in men and 18 to 32% in women, so that greater than 22% fat in males and 32% in females is considered obese. While there are several methods for accurately assessing total body fat (underwater weighting, MRI), they are expensive. A more practical approach in the clinical setting is measurement of Body Mass Index (BMI).

BODY MASS INDEX (BMI)

The BMI defined by body weight (kg) divided by height squared (m^2), was proposed by Keys as an index of relative weight and obesity. (NOTE: 1 meter = 39.3 inches, 1 kilogram = 2.2 pounds). The National Institutes of Health and the National Heart, Lung and Blood Institutes Expert Panel on Obesity suggest that BMI provides the most accurate and clinically relevant assessment of obesity.

BMI CALCULATION

BMI calculations can be made in two ways:

A. $$\text{BMI (body mass index)} = \frac{\text{weight (kg)}}{\text{height } (m^2)}$$

B. $$\text{BMI} = \frac{703 \text{ x weight in pounds}}{(\text{height in inches})^2}$$

BMI CLASSIFICATION

Weigh status	BMI (kg/m²)
Underweight	< 18.5
Normal	18.5 – 24.9
Overweight	25.0 – 29.9
Obese	30.0 – 39.9
Morbidly Obese	> 40

HEREDITY AND ENVIRONMENT

Data on the contribution of genetics to the development of human obesity vary. In adoption studies, the variance is 10 to 30%. In twin studies, it is 40 to 80%. On an average, the contribution of genetics is 25 to 40%. While genetics plays a large part in determining a person's weight, the environment also plays an important part. Although a person cannot change his or her genes, lots can be done to change the environmental component to aid with weight loss or prevent further weight gain.

Individuals vary greatly in both resting energy expenditure and activity patterns. Factors that affect energy expenditure include age and muscle mass. Therefore, a prescription of a given amount of Caloric intake calculated on the basis of energy expenditure can be incorrect for some people. The diet prescription is a trial and error process, with changes being made according to the response of the patient.

Individuals predisposed to obesity by their genetic makeup may be more influenced by environmental eating cues. Americans get about 34% of its daily Calories from fat. A high-fat diet is Calorically dense and enhances palatability, as does a high-sugar diet. Increased palatability may contribute to positive energy balance in many people.

The relative rates of obesity in the Pima Indian population of Arizona and Mexico give a good example of the interactions of genetics and environment. The Pimas, who migrated to northern Mexico many years ago, separated from the Pimas still in Arizona. The genetic makeup of the two groups is very similar. Their weights, however, are different. The Pimas in Arizona are much heavier than those in Mexico. However, their environments are very different. The Pimas in Mexico are agriculturists, active, and have no motorized equipment. They eat a diet high in carbohydrates and low in fat. The Pimas in Arizona are sedentary. They drive cars and trucks and they eat a diet high in fat, sugar, and many consume alcohol. This shows how different environments, can produce differences in weight of genetically identical groups [19, 83].

RESTING AND BASAL METABOLIC RATES (RMR AND BMR)

There is a fine distinction between RMR and BMR. RMR may be considered equal to BMR if the measurements are made in postabsorptive states. The RMR per unit body weight is not constant with age because the proportion of muscle to no muscle changes during life cycle. Adipose tissue has the lowest metabolic rate, which accounts for only 4% of the whole body RMR in non-obese individuals. This rate can increase significantly in obese people. The RMR is lower in men because they have higher muscle mass.

Study conducted among Pima Indians in Arizona indicated that persons with low RMR category had the greatest incidence of weight gain over the 4-year follow up period, while those in the high RMR group had the lowest incidence of weight gain.

Thyroid hormones play a role in regulating resting metabolism. Hyperthyroid patients have an increased metabolic rate. Hypothyroidism leads to weight gain in some people. RMR range widely even among people with normal function. Addition of thyroid hormone to weight loss programs results in excess losses of lean body mass and fat.

LEPTIN

Leptin was first identified as the protein missing in the obese mouse (ob/ob), with resulting hyperphagia, diminished energy expenditure, and increased adiposity. Leptin administration to ob/ob mice appeared to correct most abnormalities and lower body weight. These observations initially raised hopes that some human obesity occurred for similar reasons and could be treated in the same way. Nearly all studies of obese humans show a strong and consistent positive relation between plasma leptin concentrations and adipose mass. Leptin overproduction is a defect in the leptin receptor, such as in diabetic mice (db/db) but leptin receptor defects are unlikely to account for more than a small number of human cases of obesity. Therefore, current research aims to understand the role of leptin in mechanisms regulating appetite and body weight.

The leptin receptor is expressed in hypothalamic regions known to be involved in feeding behavior. Leptin receptors and neuropeptide Y cell bodies are both found in the arcuate nucleus of the hypothalamus. Because leptin decreases feeding and increases energy expenditure whereas neuropeptide Y does the opposite, several investigators have suggested that leptin may affect energy balance by altering neuropeptide Y signaling pathways. Recent data confirm that one important way leptin affects energy homeostatis is by decreasing neuropeptide Y biosynthesis in the arcuate nucleus.

One hypothesis about leptin function is that leptin provides information about the size of body fat stored to regulatory mechanisms in the brain.

That hypothesis has to be tempered by many reports showing that serum leptin concentrations are reduced by food deprivation. Leptin concentrations decrease after a 2-3 days fast or very low energy intakes from 7 days to as long as 3 months. In these situations, leptin concentrations are disproportionate to changes in adiposity.

Leptin is a regulator that is missing from obese mice, whereas concentration are elevated in most obese humans, and it reflects adiposity during a weight-stable period, but does not reflect adiposity during a period of food restriction. It appears likely that the changed state of energy balance is a key variable. When energy balance is in steady state, leptin concentrations correlate well with the amount of adipose tissue. Significant changes in energy balance with non-steady state conditions, particularly total-body energy loss, appear to decrease serum leptin out of proportion to changes in fat mass.

A variety of hormones, regulators, and metabolites change quickly during periods of either acute food deprivation or chronic food restriction. For example, serum cholesterol concentrations drop with food restriction, before major decreases in body weight occur. Similar changes occur in insulin, thyroid hormone, blood pressure, and a variety of constitutive proteins with short half-lives. Sympathetic nervous activity is also diminished during energy deprivation. Thus, leptin may be responding as other proteins do to the energy status of the individual, which eventually is reflected in body weight. It is also possible that leptin secretion from adipose cells is in part regulated by other factors such as the sympathetic nervous system, insulin, or glucocorticoids. It is suggested that the hexosamine biosynthetic pathway may serve as a nutrient sensor that regulates leptin gene expression in muscle and fat. The end product of this pathway, UDP-N-acetylglucosamine, results in rapid and marked increases in leptin messenger RNA and protein. Also, leptin synthesis is stimulated with hyperglycemia or hyperipidemia, which also increases concentrations of UDP-N-acetylglucosamine in rodents. Thus, leptin concentrations may be influenced by a nutrient sensing mechanism, rather than being a simple reflection of total body adiposity [60, 71, 86, 92].

BINGE EATING

Binge eating is a distinct eating pattern in some obese individuals. Binge eating is the consumption of large amounts of food in short periods of time. Binge eaters closely resemble normal-weight bulimia nervosa patients with the exception that obese individuals do not have binging behavior. Binge eaters ingest significantly more than non-binge eaters of comparable body weight. Binge eaters consume more fat during binge episodes. Obese binge eaters have higher rates of mood disorder than obese non-binge eaters.

The relationship between binge eating and obesity is very complex. We don't know whether binge eating causes obesity or obesity causes binge eating.

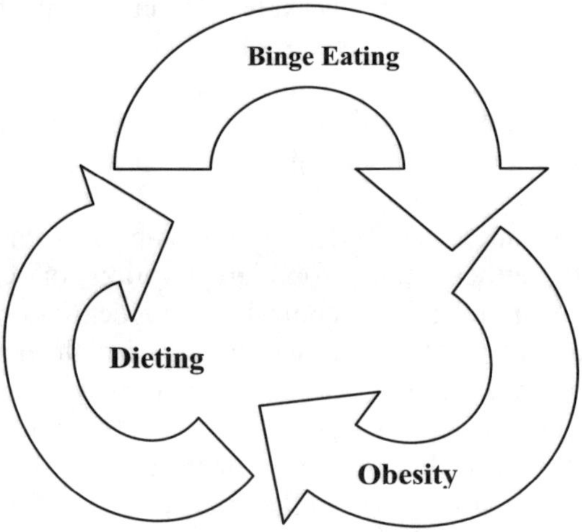

Persons with binge eating problems who are overweight may lose some weight but loss may be very slow and not as great as they would like. Repeated cycles of weight loss and regain, sometimes called "yo-yo" dieting, may change body composition and metabolism in ways that make subsequent attempts to lose weight more difficult [82, 183].

OVERCOMING BINGE EATING

1. Recording in detail all eating at the time it occurs, together with thoughts and feelings.
2. Introducing regular eating plan. This will displace many binges.
3. Using alternative behavior to help resist urges to binge eating.
4. Introducing avoided foods into the diet.
5. Gradually eliminating other forms of strict dieting.
6. Developing skills to deal with problems that might trigger binges.

7. Considering the role of family and social factors.
8. Drawing up a plan for dealing with any future difficulties.

STEPS TO INTRODUCE A PATTERN OF REGULAR EATING

Aim should be to eat three planned meals and snacks each day. A typical plan would be:

- Breakfast
- Mid-morning snack
- Lunch
- Mid-afternoon snack
- Dinner
- Evening snack

Additionally:

1. Eating should be dictated by preset plan and not by sensation of hunger.
2. Do not leave more than four hours between planned meals and snacks.
3. Do not skip meals or snack.
4. Do not eat between the planned meals and snacks.
5. If binge occurs between meals and snacks, it is important to get on track as soon as possible.
6. At the beginning of each day, work out the times you are going to eat.
7. Keep a food diary.
8. Restrict eating to certain places in home.

WAIST CIRCUMFERENCE

Excess abdominal fat is an important risk factor. The evaluation of waist circumference to assess the risk associated with cardiovascular disease (CVD) is supported by research. Research has shown that a person who has excess fact in the lower body (gluteofemoral area) will have a lower health risk than a person with excess fat in the abdomen and upper truncal area. Since more men than women tend to put on excess weight in the abdomen, men are at greater risk. While the most accurate way to measure central obesity is by magnetic resonance imaging (MRI) or computed tomography (CT) scanning, these are too expensive for routine use. As a result, simple anthropometric measurements like the waist circumference measurement or the waist-to-hip ratio (WHR) can be made. Above 100 cm (30 inches) is abnormal for the waist measurement; for WHR, a value above 0.85 for women and above 1.0 for men indicates increased health risk.

There is no relationship between total body fatness and abdominal distribution of fat. BMI alone is not a good predictor of the level of abdominal fat. It is for this reason that additional measures of regional fat distribution are used, such as waist circumference, waist-to-hip ratio, waist-to-thigh ratio, or more recently, waist-to-height ratio. Interaction of obesity with excess abdominal fat leads to metabolic complications. As BMI values increase above 25, a high WHR is associated with increasing health risk. A person who has a BMI of 35 and a WHR of 1.0 will have a much greater abdominal adipose tissue mass than one with a comparable WHR but a BMI of 25. Therefore, both the degree of obesity and the distribution must be considered in the assessment of disease risk.

OTHER REGIONAL FAT DISTRIBUTION

Subcutaneous skinfold measurement is used to assess body fat distribution. The most common measurements for peripheral fat are the triceps, biceps and thigh. Ratios of central-to-peripheral skinfold are sometimes used.

In everyday practice, it may not be practical for the physician to make all those measurements. The recommended measurements include:

1. Weight
2. Height
3. Waist circumference
4. Hip circumference
5. Waist/Hip Ratio (WHR)
6. Body Mass Index (see the appendix)

EVIDENCE FOR SUCCESS OF CALORIC RESTRICTION IN WEIGHT LOSS AND CONTROL

American adults utilize many methods in an attempt to lose weight, including consuming low-calorie foods and beverages, using exercise, attending weight loss classes, taking medication, using meal substitutions, or skipping meals. In a survey from the Calorie Control Council, 97% of American dieters reduced their intake of high-calorie foods as a means of losing weight and maintaining weight loss. Given that 24% of American men and 36% of American women are currently trying to lose weight, the topic of success in weight loss and maintenance programs is usually the quantity of pounds reduced and loss maintained. Calorie restriction and other features of a weight loss program may have association with its various adverse health effects that are also important to consider. Therefore, successful weight loss programs need to be presented to the public in a manner in which safety is a paramount factor. The more aggressive programs often require close medical supervision.

In an attempt to gather data from industry addressing the issue of efficacy and safety associated with weight loss. Data was gathered on weight loss products to provide any data they might have on success of various programs for weight loss, targeted for use by the average overweight person, or designed for treatment of morbid obesity. There were various plans, including 60 reprints of peer-reviewed articles. Information was provided by the makers of three nonphysician-directed weight loss programs and two physician-directed programs.

They reviewed the data with three primary considerations in mind:

1) What is the evidence that current practices of weight control are safe and effective?
2) How representative are the data with respect to products used by the average overweight US citizen?
3) How do the various products and plans that are marketed position themselves as normal food, food for special dietary use, or medical food (restricted to use under physician care)?

FRUCTOSE AND OBESITY

The consumption of high-fructose corn syrup (HFCS) has increased. However, HFCS as is, is not composed predominantly of fructose as the name implies. The two most widely used forms of HFCS in the United States contain either 42% or 55% fructose with the remainder being mostly glucose. Table sugar (sucrose) is a 50-50 mixture of these two components. Both HFCS and table sugar have the same number of calories on a dry weight basis. Because HFCS and table sugar are so similar, the two sweeteners can be used interchangeably without having a substantial effect on the diet.

There has not been a dramatic increase in the intake of fructose compared to other simple sugars in the United States. The use of HFCS as a sweetener in US foods and beverages (including soft drinks) has increased dramatically during the past 30 years because it has a sweet taste, it costs less than sugar. Sugar use decreased from 83% of all sweeteners used in 1970 to 43% in 1997 while HFCS increased from 16 to 56% during the same period. However, this marked shift in sweetener usage had not had a major impact on the fructose content of the US diet because HFCS and sucrose have similar compositions. There is no credible scientific evidence to justify signaling out HFCS as a unique contributor to obesity.

The body cannot distinguish between fructose from HFCS or any other source. Carbohydrates are broken down into their individual sugar molecules by the digestive system before absorbed into the bloodstream. Once absorbed, the body has no way of knowing whether a molecule of fructose came from sucrose, HFCS, honey or fruit. Since the proportion of glucose and fructose in HFCS and sucrose are similar, these two sweeteners are virtually indistinguishable by the body.

Unlike glucose, fructose has a very low glycemic index and does not cause the body to produce large amounts of insulin. Insulin is well known for its ability to enable the body to use glucose, but it also depresses appetite. In addition, prolonged exposure to insulin causes the brain to synthesize the hormone leptin, which is believed to decrease food intake on a long-term basis. It is possible, that diets very high in fructose could predispose to obesity because the regulatory mechanisms designed to control food intake may not be fully functional. In addition, unlike glucose and other simple sugars, fructose enters the metabolic pathway downstream from a control point that helps regulate the synthesis of fat.

Human studies suggest that usual intakes of fructose do not increase risk of obesity. Human volunteers who consumed calorie-controlled diets containing a high-fructose meal replacement product (~50% of carbohydrate as fructose) lost just as much weight after 12 weeks as subjects who consumed a similar product in which all of the carbohydrate came from glucose.

The metabolic rate and storage of body fat was identical among obese and lean women who were fed diets with 50% excess calories from fat, sucrose, glucose, or fructose.

The intake of HFCS has remained very low in Europe during the past 15 years. But the incidence of obesity has increased significantly.

A calorie is a calorie. There are no long-term human studies designed to determine the effect of feeding fructose on body weight. Nevertheless, the recent studies cited above suggest that a calorie from fructose is no different than a calorie from glucose or any other sugar with respect to body weight.

Obesity is caused by too many calories and not enough physical activity – not fructose, sucrose, soft drinks or any single food. The key to maintaining a healthy body weight is eating a diet based on balance, variety and moderation along with regular physical activity.

FAST FOODS

Fast foods present the greatest risks to the health of Americans. These foods are high in total fat, saturated fat, cholesterol, sodium, and are very low in fiber. It has been shown that 1/3 of Americans consume 45% of their daily energy from junk foods. High fat junk foods are displacing healthier foods and causing the epidemic of obesity. (Chapter 10)

PHYSICAL ACTIVITY

Lack of exercise is a big contributor to obesity. Energy expenditure must equal food intake. (Details are in Chapter 6).

Chapter 5

HEALTH RISKS OF OBESITY

Persons with obesity are at risk of developing one or more serious medical conditions. Obesity is associated with more than 30 medical conditions, and scientific research has shown a strong relationship with at least 15 of these conditions. A weight loss of 10% in overweight and obese persons can improve medical conditions related to obesity [72-74, 89].

Prevalence of various medical conditions for men and women are shown in Tables 1 and 2.

TABLE 1
Prevalence of Medical Conditions by Body Mass Index (BMI) for Men

Medical Condition	Body Mass Index			
	18.5-24.9	25-29.9	30-34.9	> 40
	Prevalence (%)			
Type 2 Diabetes	2.03	4.93	10.10	10.65
Coronary Heart Disease	8.84	9.60	16.01	13.97
High Blood Pressure	23.47	34.16	48.95	64.53
Osteoarthritis	2.59	4.55	4.66	10.04

Source: *NHANES III, 1988 – 1994*

FACTS ABOUT OBESITY AND MEDICAL CONDITIONS

Arthritis

Osteoarthritis (OA)

- Obesity is associated with the development of OA of the hand, hip, back, and especially the knee as shown in Tables 1 and 2.
- At a Body Mass Index (BMI) of > 25, the incidence of OA has been shown to steadily increase.
- Modest weight loss of 10 to 15 pounds is likely to relieve symptoms and delay disease progression of knee OA.

TABLE 2
Prevalence of Medical Conditions by Body Mass Index (BMI) for Women

Medical Condition	Body Mass Index			
	18.5-24.9	25-29.9	30-34.9	> 40
	Prevalence (%)			
Type 2 Diabetes	2.38	7.12	7.24	19.89
Coronary Heart Disease	6.87	11.13	12.56	19.22
High Blood Pressure	23.26	38.77	47.95	63.16
Osteoarthritis	5.22	8.51	9.94	17.19

Source: *NHANES III, 1988 – 1994*

Rheumatoid Arthritis (RA)

- Obesity has been found to be related to RA in both men and women.

Birth Defects

- Maternal obesity (BMI > 29) has been associated with an increase in incidence of neural tube defects (NTD) in several studies. Variable results have been found in this area.
- Folate intake, which decreases the risk of NTD's, was found in one study to have a reduced effect with higher pre-pregnancy weight.

Cancers

Breast Cancer

- Postmenopausal women with obesity have a higher risk of developing breast cancer. Weight gain after menopause may also increase breast cancer risk.
- Women who gain about 45 pounds or more after age 18 are twice as likely to develop breast cancer after menopause than those who remain weight stable.
- Premenopausal women diagnosed with breast cancer who are overweight appear to have a shorter life span than women with lower BMI.
- The risk of breast cancer in men is also increased by obesity.

Cancers of the Esophagus and Stomach Gardia

- Obesity is strongly associated with cancer of the esophagus and the risk becomes higher with increasing BMI.
- The risk for gastric cancer rises moderately with increasing BMI.

Colorectal Cancer

- High BMI, high Calorie intake, and low physical activity are independent risk factors of colorectal cancer.
- Larger waist size (abdominal obesity) is associated with colorectal cancer.

Endometrial Cancer (EC)

- Women with obesity have three to four times the risk of EC than women with lower BMI.
- Women with obesity and diabetes are reported to have a 3-fold increase in risk for EC above the risk of obesity alone.
- Body size is a risk factor for EC regardless of where fat is distributed in the body.

Renal Cell Cancer

- Consistent evidence has been found to associate obesity with renal cell cancer, especially in women.
- Excess weight was reported in one study to account for 21% of renal cell cancer cases.

Cardiovascular Disease (CVD)

- Obesity increases CVD risk due to its effect on blood lipid levels as shown in Tables 1 and 2.
- Weight loss improves blood lipid levels by lowering triglycerides and LDL ("bad") cholesterol and increasing HDL ("good") cholesterol.
- Weight loss of 5% to 10% can reduce total blood cholesterol.
- The effects of obesity on cardiovascular health can begin in childhood, which increases the risk of developing CVD as an adult.
- Overweight and obesity increase the risk of illness and death associated with coronary heart disease.
- Obesity is a major risk factor for heart attack, and is now recognized as such by the American Heart Association.

Carpal Tunnel Syndrome (CTS)

- Obesity has been established as a risk factor for CTS.
- The odds of an obese patient having CTS were found in one study to be almost four times greater than that of a non-obese patient.
- Seventy percent of persons in a recent CTS study were overweight or obese.

Chronic Venous Insufficiency (CVI)

- Patients with CVI, inadequate blood flow through the veins, tend to be older, male, and have obesity.

Daytime Sleepiness

- People with obesity frequently complain of daytime sleepiness and fatigue, two probable causes of mass transportation accidents.
- Severe obesity has been associated with increased daytime sleepiness even in the absence of sleep apnea or other breathing disorders.

Deep Vein Thrombosis (DVT)

- Obesity increases the risk of DVT, a condition that disrupts the normal process of blood clotting.
- Patients with obesity have an increased risk of DVT after surgery.

Diabetes (Type 2)

- Approximately 90% of individuals with type 2 diabetes are reported to be overweight or obese.
- Obesity has been found to be the largest environmental influence on the prevalence of diabetes in a population.
- Obesity complicates the management of type 2 diabetes by increasing insulin resistance and glucose intolerance, which makes drug treatment for type 2 diabetes less effective.
- A weight loss of as little as 5% can reduce high blood sugar.

End Stage Renal Disease (ESRD)

- Obesity may be a direct or indirect factor in the initiation or progression of renal disease, as suggested in preliminary data.

Gallbladder Disease

- Obesity is an established predictor of gallbladder disease.
- Obesity and rapid weight loss in obese persons are known risk factors for gallstones.
- Gallstones are common among overweight and obese persons. Gallstones appear in persons who are obese, at a rate of 30% versus 10% in non-obese.

Gout

- Obesity contributes to the cause of gout – the deposit of uric acid crystals in joints and tissue.
- Obesity is associated with increased production of uric acid and decreased elimination from the body.

Heart Disorders

- Obesity has been found to be a risk factor for heart condition.

Hypertension

- Over 75% of hypertension cases are reported to be directly attributed to obesity.
- Weight or BMI in association with age is the strongest indicator of blood pressure in humans.
- The association between obesity and high blood pressure has been observed in virtually all societies, ages, ethnic groups, and in both genders.
- The risk of developing hypertension is five to six times greater in obese adult Americans, age 20 to 45, compared to non-obese individuals of the same age.

Impaired Immune Response

- Obesity has been found to decrease the body's resistance to harmful organisms.
- A decrease in the activity of scavenger cells, that destroy bacteria and foreign organisms in the body, has been observed in patients with obesity.

Impaired Respiratory Function

- Obesity is associated with impairment in respiratory function.
- Obesity has been found to increase respiratory resistance, which in turn may cause breathlessness.

- Decreases in lung volume with increasing obesity have been reported.

Infections Following Wounds

- Obesity is associated with the increased incidence of wound infection.
- Burn patients with obesity are reported to develop pneumonia and wound infection with twice the frequency of non-obese.

Infertility

- Obesity increases the risk for several reproductive disorders, negatively affecting normal menstrual function and fertility.
- Loss of about 10% of initial weight is effective in improving menstrual regularity, ovulation, hormonal profiles and pregnancy rates.

Liver Disease

- Excess weight is reported to be an independent risk factor for the development of alcohol related liver diseases including cirrhosis and acute hepatitis.
- Obesity is the most common factor of nonalcoholic steato-hepatitis, a major cause of progressive liver disease.

Low Back Pain

- Obesity may play a part in aggravating a simple low back problem, and contribute to a long-lasting or recurring condition
- Women who are overweight or have a large waist size are reported to be particularly at risk for low back pain.

Obstetric and Gynecologic Complications

- Women with severe obesity have a menstrual disturbance rate three times higher than that of women with normal weight.
- High pre-pregnancy weight is associated with an increased risk during pregnancy of hypertension, gestational diabetes, urinary infection, Cesarean section and toxemia.
- Obesity is reportedly associated with the increased incidence of overdue births, induced labor and longer labors.
- Women with maternal obesity have more cesarean deliveries and higher incidence of blood loss during delivery as well as infection and wound complication after surgery.

- Complications after childbirth associated with obesity include an increased risk of endometrial infection and inflammation, urinary tract infection, and urinary incontinence.

Pain

- Bodily pain is a prevalent problem among persons with obesity.
- Greater disability due to bodily pain has been reported by persons with obesity compared to persons with other chronic medical conditions.
- Obesity is known to be associated with musculoskeletal or joint-related pain.
- Foot pain located at the heel, known as Sever's disease is commonly associated with obesity.

Pancreatitis

- Obesity is a predictive factor of outcome in acute pancreatitis.
- Obese patients with acute pancreatitis are reported to develop significantly more complications, including respiratory failure, than non-obese.
- Patients with severe pancreatitis have been found to have a higher body-fat percentage and larger waist size than patients with mild pancreatitis.

Sleep Apnea

- Obesity, particularly upper body obesity, is the most significant risk factor for obstructive sleep apnea.
- There is a 12 to 30-fold higher incidence of obstructive sleep apnea among morbidly obese patients compared to the general population.
- Among patients with obstructive sleep apnea, at least 60% to 70% are obese.

Stroke

- Elevated BMI is reported to increase the risk of ischemic stroke independent of other risk factors including age and systolic blood pressure.
- Abdominal obesity appears to predict the risk of stroke in men.
- Obesity and weight gain are risk factors for ischemic and total stroke in women.

Surgical Complications

- Obesity is a risk factor for complications after a surgery.
- Surgical patients with obesity demonstrate a higher number of incidences of hospital-acquired infections compared to normal weight patients.

Urinary Stress Incontinence

- Obesity is a well-documented risk factor for urinary stress incontinence, involuntary urine loss, as well as urge incontinence and urgency among women.
- Obesity is reported to be a strong risk factor for several urinary symptoms after pregnancy and delivery, continuing as much as 6 to 18 months after childbirth.

Other Conditions

- Several other obesity-related conditions have been reported by various researchers including:

  Abdominal hernias, acanthosis nigricans, endocrine abnormallities, chronic hypoxia and hypercapnia, dermatological effects, depression, elephantitis, gastroesophageal reflux, heel spurs, hirsutism, lower extremity edema, mammegaly (causing considerable problems such as bra strap pain, skin damage, cervical pain, chronic odors and infections in the skin folds under the breasts, etc.), large anterior abdominal wall masses (abdominal paniculitis with frequent panniculitis, impeding walking, causing frequent infections, odors, clothing difficulties, low back pain), musculoskeletal disease, prostate cancer, pseudo tumor cerebri (or benign intracranial hypertension), and sliding hiatil hernia.

Source: *American Obesity Association (AOA). These fact sheets are a product of AOA's National Campaign of Obesity Education, instituted to provide current information on obesity based on scientific evidence.*

THE OBESITY-DIABETES CONNECTION: MANAGEMENT OF OBESE TYPE II DIABETES

Diabetes is the most prevalent endocrine disease in humans. It is a group of clinical syndromes that exhibit insulin intolerance. Type II diabetes or non-insulin dependent diabetes mellitus (NIDDM) accounts for approximately 90% of all cases of diabetes and it is present in 3% of the US population (Figure 1, Tables 1 – 4). There is estimated to be almost an equal number of undiagnosed cases of NIDDM.

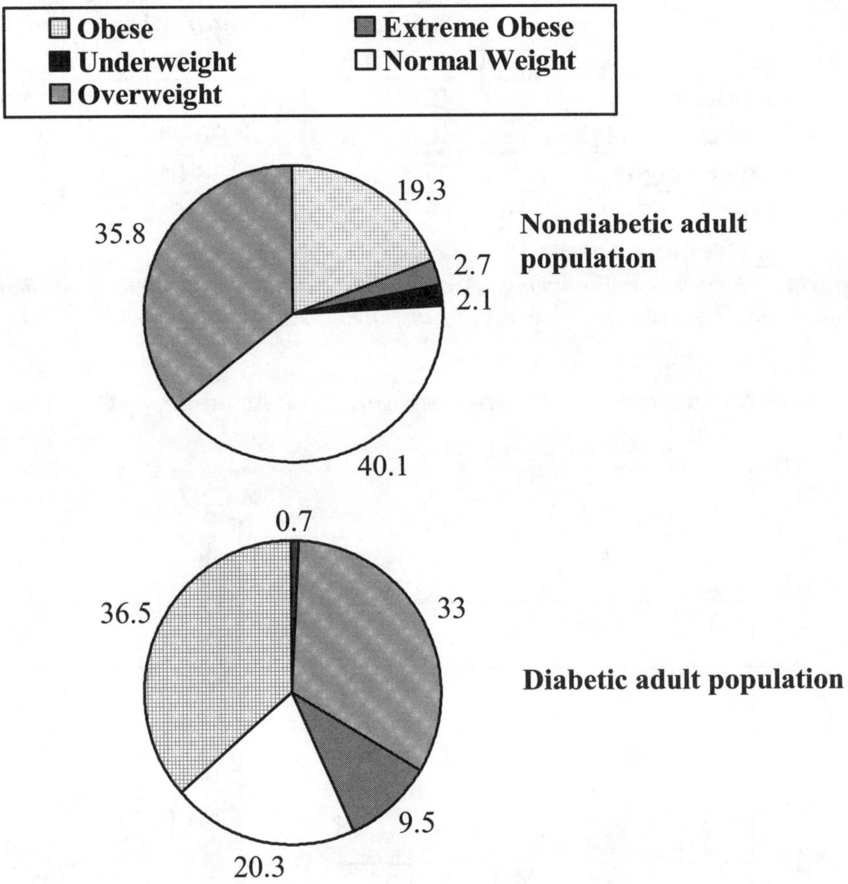

FIGURE 1

Percentage distribution of nondiabetic (top) and diabetic (bottom) adults in the US community population, by BMI status, 2001
Source: *Center for Financing, Access and Cost Trends, AHRQ, Medical Expenditure Panel Survey-Household Component, 2001*

TABLE 3

Percentage distribution of nondiabetic and diabetic in the US community 2001

	Nondiabetic Adult Population	Diabetic Adult Population
Underweight	2.1%	0.7%
Normal Weight	40.1%	20.3%
Overweight	35.8%	33.0%
Obese	19.3%	36.5%
Extremely Obese	2.7%	9.5%

Source: *Center for Financing, Access, and Cost Trends, AHRQ, Medical Expenditure Panel Survey-Household Component, 2001.*

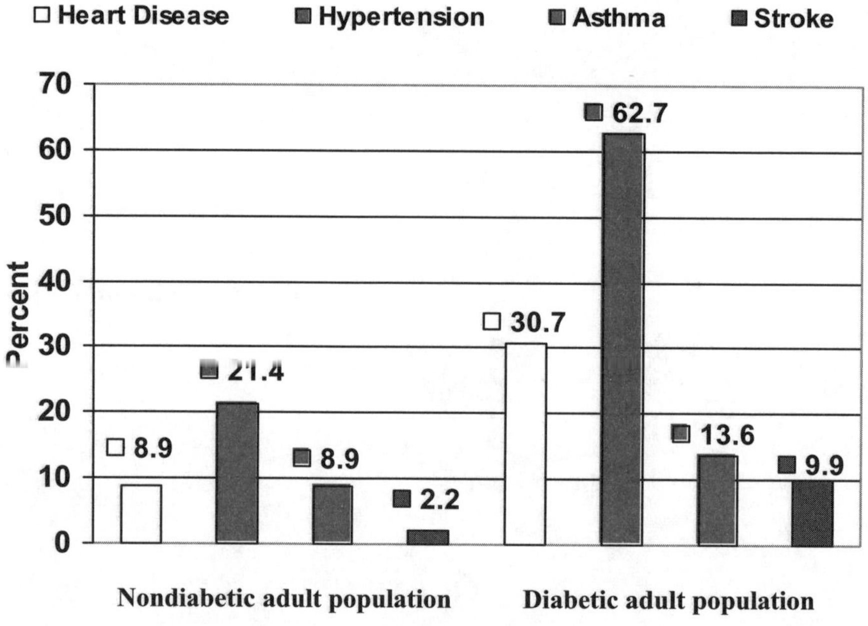

FIGURE 2

Percentage of nondiabetic and diabetic adults in the US community population with selected health conditions, 2001

Source: *Center for Financing, Access and Cost Trends, AHRQ, Medical Expenditure Panel Survey-Household Component, 2001*

TABLE 4
Percentage distribution of some chronic diseases among nondiabetic and diabetic adults in the US (2001)

	Nondiabetic Adult Population	Diabetic Adult Population
Heart Disease	8.9%	30.7%
Hypertension	21.4%	62.7%
Asthma	8.9%	13.6%
Stroke	2.2%	9.9%

Source: *Center for Financing, Access, and Cost Trends, AHRQ, Medical Expenditure Panel Survey-Household Component, 2001*

Figure 1 and Table 3 show that 19 percent nondiabetics were obese as opposed to 37 percent obese diabetic. Figure 2 and Table 4 show that heart disease, hypertension, asthma and stroke were higher in diabetic adult population.

NIDDM is a somewhat neglected disorder because it is a milder form of diabetes compared to type I. Most patients seem asymptomatic, and metabolic disorders such as acute hyperglycemia are rare.

Insulin resistance that characterizes type II diabetes can be either as a result of a lack of insulin receptors, or insufficient amount of insulin, and this results in hyperglycemia. This insulin resistance is associated with an increase in body weight. In obese individuals, the hyperglycemia is more severe compared to non-obese individuals with NIDDM. Most type II diabetics are either obese or overweight, and they account for approximately 90% of the diagnosed cases of diabetes mellitus. Even so, it is not until recently that this link between obesity and type II diabetes has been understood. Even moderate obesity, particularly abdominal obesity can increase the risk for NIDDM almost ten-fold.

The mechanism by which obesity causes diabetes has been determined at the molecular level. This insulin resistance is mainly thought to be due to defects in the insulin-responsive glucose-transport system, and in particular the decline in the number or activity of glucose transporter molecules. In obese individuals, the adipose tissue produces vast amounts of the cytokine tumor necrosis factor-alpha. This cytokine inhibits the synthesis of a protein called glut-4. The glut-4 is a glucose transporter that translocates glucose across the plasma membrane when insulin is bound to the insulin receptor. Cells cannot take up glucose when glut-4 is not present, and this explains the resistance to insulin.

The major health risks of obesity increase when the weight gain begins in adulthood and continue for many years. These individuals have twice the risk of developing diabetes. NIDDM is mostly found in people over the age of forty.

There is a strong genetic linkage related to NIDDM. In fact, more than 90% of monozygotic twins would both develop NIDDM, and the offspring of parents that have NIDDM have a 35% risk of getting the disease. Most of the patients that have a family history of NIDDM are obese. Thus genetic predisposition plays an important role in obesity. However this does not mean that a person with a family history of obesity is destined to become obese regardless of his or her dietary and physical activity habits. Thus primary care providers should caution close family members, especially first-degree relatives, to avoid obesity, make appropriate adjustments to diet and engage in physical activity. Even modest weight reduction could be beneficial for individuals with elevated waist-to-hip ratios, regardless of whether they are obese or not.

Controlling obesity is the primary method of both preventing the onset of type II diabetes, as well as lessening the hyperglycemic effects of diabetes in cases where diabetes is already present.

Treatment for type II diabetics should concentrate on preventive measures that would postpone as long as possible the need for antidiabetic medications. The American Diabetes Association guidelines for medical nutrition therapy for diabetes mellitus are to achieve a normal metabolic control, and to prevent medical complications of diabetes. The NIH report on overweight and obesity shows that there are three principle guidelines to be followed. These are the prevention of weight gain, weight loss, as well as maintenance of weight loss.

The prevention of weight gain is targeted to those individuals who may not be willing to do what it takes to lose weight. Therefore the maintenance of their current weight is a better alternative compared to them gaining any more weight. It is normally difficult for the healthcare providers to identify these individuals. However there could be indicators such as refusing counseling from a dietitian, failing to maintain a log of meals eaten, and other similar situations. Other factors could create negative attitudes towards exercise and physical activity, lack of awareness of health risks involved, as well as lack of family or social support.

Weight loss is for the motivated patient who would be willing to follow the guideline for losing weight. The NIH recommends that obese individuals should attempt to lose approximately 10% of their body weight over a period of 6 months. This is possible with a reduction in daily caloric intake as well as an increase in the basal metabolic rate to burn off more energy. For individuals with BMI 25-35, the caloric deficit should be 300-500 kcal per day, and the average weight loss should be almost one pound. For individuals with BMI over 35, the caloric deficit should be between 500-1000 kcal per day, and the weight loss should average almost 2 pounds per week.

Weight maintenance is defined by the NIH as less than 6.6 pounds weight gain and a sustained reduction in waist circumference of four inches over a 24-month period (NIH, 2001) enough to offset the metabolic effects brought on by obesity even though the individual is still obese.

The methods of losing weight are diet therapy, physical activity, behavioral therapy, and anti-obesity drugs. Also dietary management is imperative if insulin sensitivity is to be improved. The dietary therapy includes a Caloric deficit of 250-1000 kcal per day with a healthy balanced diet. A registered dietitian is the best person to implement such therapy. Lists that tell the patient what to avoid are normally not recommended because they are unrealistic as a guideline for the patient to follow. This would create another barrier for the patient who is already overwhelmed by the pressure of losing weight. The diet should vary according to each patient and should not be a complete deprivation from the type of food that they are used to. Most importantly, the diet therapy should result in achieving a desirable body weight just as in any normal healthy individual. It has been estimated that a reduction in Caloric intake by approximately 500 kcal per day less than the requirement for weight maintenance should result in a loss between one and 2 kg per month.

The diet is designed to keep blood sugar and lipids within normal levels. The American Diabetes Association recommends that the diet for weight loss should include fat content of not more than 30% of caloric intake, carbohydrates of 55% or more, and proteins should make up the rest of the requirements. Both saturated fats and cholesterol should be restricted, while the diet should encourage intake of monounsaturated fats. The Caloric requirements of a diabetic are the same as those for a normal individual, and these should not be compromised at the expense of a strict diet. When it is desirable to lose a large amount of weight, as is the case with these patients, it is better to set short-term goals.

Another important and mostly overlooked component of dietary therapy is educating the patient on diet. This education should entail teaching the patient how to read food labels and healthy ways of cooking food. Management of caloric requirements improves glycemic control as well as insulin sensitivity, regardless of the amount of weight loss, especially in these obese patients with NIDDM. Dietary management should result in a NIDDM patient with a higher life expectancy and normal health.

Physical activity is very important in the prevention and treatment of diabetes. In addition to diet therapy, exercise is the best method for long-term weight control. Normally this entails a major change in the lifestyle of the obese individual and also needs a lot of discipline. It is important that the patient understands that exercise alone may not be sufficient, and that controlling Caloric intake may be more important in losing weight. A number of studies have shown that exercise enhances weight loss, but only to a maximum of 3 kg. It is important that the patient is aware of this so that he or she does not get discouraged. However, exercise sustains weight loss more effectively than diet alone. Patients on a diet who do not exercise regularly have been shown to gain back the weight they have lost.

Even if the patient does not lose weight from exercise, there is improved glycemic control. This is mainly due to improvement in the action of insulin on uptake of glucose in muscle. Also insulin levels have been shown to either stay constant or even decrease during exercise, suggesting that exercise may actually improve insulin sensitivity. Heavy exercise increases muscle mass and thus increases the area over which insulin can function effectively.

The level of exercise should vary according to the patient because some patients may have other underlying problems and cardiovascular risk should be assessed. In a NIDDM patient without a heart condition, an exercise tolerance test may be sufficient. Then a moderate exercise program can be followed so that the patient does not get discouraged. This should vary according to the patient. Once the patient is comfortable with this exercise program, more intense exercises can be added over a period of a few weeks. This should not be restricted and should include recreational activity, as well as other daily activities that the patient would otherwise not engage before. The key is encouragement and gradual improvement.

HIGH FIBER AND GLYCEMIC INDEX

While concern exists about the practicality of following a diet significantly high in fiber or eating a diet consisting primarily of low glycemic response foods, the health benefits seen in lowering lipid levels, blood pressure, blood glucose and prevention of cancer are great. These are two additional lifestyle modification techniques that can be utilized with patients who have an interest in improving their health.

FIBER

Fiber is only obtained from plant products not animal products as discussed earlier. The foods that contain fiber are grains, fruits and vegetables. The current American diet is estimated to contain 10-20 grams of fiber per day. The recommendation given by the American Diabetes Association is a modest increase to 20-35 grams of fiber per day. It has been reported that 50 grams of fiber per day has noted health benefits.

Soluble fiber dissolves in water but more importantly it absorbs water as it is very viscous. This is the type of fiber that the most benefit has been seen in regard to lowering lipid levels and glucose. Foods higher in soluble fiber and resistant to gelatinization slow the rate of digestion and absorption. Examples of soluble fiber are: legumes (beans, peas), lentils, and oat bran, and some fruits and vegetables [35].

GLYCEMIC INDEX

The Glycemic Index ranks carbohydrate containing foods according to the glycemic response or impact of that food on post-prandial blood glucose as compared to a reference food, either being glucose or white bread. Low glycemic foods cause a small rise in blood glucose and high glycemic foods cause a significant rise in blood glucose post-prandially. A Glycemic Index has been created utilizing this information. The scale runs from 0 to 100 [28].

There are several factors that affect the glycemic response of food: Cooking methods and processing; particle size and gelatinization of starch granules; and fat content. The more processed a food or the smaller the particle size, the higher the glycemic response. The less processed or cooked the food, the larger the particle size, and the higher the fat content, the lower the glycemic response. There is raised concern that a high fat content of a food causes a lower glycemic response. This concern should be addressed with the patient through a discussion about better choices.

Higher glycemic response foods are refined grain products, potatoes, and refined breakfast cereals. Lower glycemic response foods are beans, peas, lentils, whole grain cereals, fruits, and vegetables. Lower glycemic response foods are also good sources of fibers. The glycemic index of foods is listed in Table 5. Among the breads, bagel has highest glycemic index.

TABLE 5
Glycemic Index (Reference food is 50 grams of glucose solution)

Bread		**Breakfast Cereal**			
Oat bran	48	All-bran	42		
Wholegrain	48	Oatmeal	49		
White	70	Cream of Wheat	70		
Bagel	72	Corn Flakes	83		
Root Vegetables		**Rice/Spaghetti**		**Fruits**	
Beans/Lentils	28	Brown rice	55	Cherries	22
Carrots	39	Spaghetti	41	Pear	37
Sweet potato	54	Wild rice	57	Apple	38
Boiled potato	56	White rice (long-grain)	58	Orange	44
Mashed potato	73			Grapes	46
French fries	75			Banana	55
Instant potato	83			Pineapple	66

SUMMARY

- Eat more whole grains, fresh fruits and fresh vegetables. This is consistent with the AHA guidelines, American Cancer Society, and American Diabetes Association guidelines for a healthy diet.

- Eat lower glycemic response foods in place of higher glycemic response foods more often. Lower glycemic response foods are whole grain bread, bran cereal, old fashioned oatmeal, barley, beans, peas, lentils, bulgur, parboiled rice, oat bran, and pasta.

- Eat less high glycemic response foods like instant rice, potatoes, refined breakfast cereals. Substitute lower glycemic response foods whenever possible.

- Eat less low glycemic response foods that are high in calories such as baked goods and ice cream.

- Follow the ADA guidelines, 50-60% Carbohydrates, 20% Protein, 25-30% Fat.

- If there is hypertriglyceredimia, consume only 40% Carbohydrates.

Table 6 provides examples of high and low glycemic meals.

TABLE 6
Examples of High and Low Glycemic Meals

	Gycemic Index	Fiber (gm)
High Glycemic Meal		
2 slices bagel	72	1
3 ounces turkey	0	0
2 tsp mayonnaise/margarine	0	0
Small banana	55	0.5
2 sugar cookies	80	1
potato chips (small bag 1&1/2 oz)	54	1
soft drink	68	0
Low Glycemic Meal		
2 slices whole grain bread	48	6
3 ounces turkey	0	0
2 tsp mayonnaise/margarine	0	0
1 whole small apple	38	2
2 oatmeal cookies	55	3
popcorn (small bag 1.5 oz)	55	5
milk, low fat	32	0

It is apparent that obesity is indeed a major health problem in this country and control of obesity would result in a major drop in the number of patients suffering from NIDDM. The link between obesity and NIDDM is clear and the best way to address the problem is to start with preventing obesity. This would entail informing people of the health risks associated with weight gain and the ways in which lifestyle changes could be beneficial [40, 45, 59, 61, 65, 85, 103].

LIVER DISEASES OF OBESITY

Obesity is the predominant cause of non-alcoholic hepatic steatosis and steatohepatitis (NASH). The exact prevalence of these hepatic disorders in obesity is unknown but is clearly underestimated by available studies. The pathogenesis of both disorders is poorly understood, but is probably a result of complex interplay of factors, including increased delivery of free fatty acids to the liver, alterations in insulin signaling, diminished mitochondrial β oxidation and increased oxidative stress. Treatment options are unsatisfactory and no treatment has been proven in clinical trials to reverse hepatic steatosis or NASH in adults. Moderate sustained weight loss is recommended [25, 43, 44, 187].

Hepatic steatosis, or fatty liver, is the accumulation of fat, usually in the form of triglyceride, within the hepatocytes [2]. This may be associated with mild inflammation. Fatty liver is the most common liver disorder in the world, but the true prevalence of hepatic steatosis in obesity is unknown. Many of the estimates of prevalence of fatty liver have been defined in selected populations, such as patients with abnormal liver function tests or patients selected for surgical therapy of obesity. In obese patients selected to undergo jejunoileal bypass, gastric bypass, or biliopancreatic diversion, fatty liver is the most common histologic lesion of the liver, and is found in 50-95% of patients. A recent study from Italy showed a prevalence of steatosis of 76% among obese nonalcoholic adults. The distribution of body fat may be more important in the development of non-alcoholic fatty liver diseases (NAFLD) than the total adipose mass. Studies have shown a significant correlation between the degree of hepatic steatosis and the waist-to-hip ratio, pointing to the importance of intraabdominal or visceral fat as a predictor of fatty liver. Fatty liver is the mildest form of NAFLD and can be caused by a number of clinical conditions and medications [15].

The epidemiology of NASH, which is a more significant histologic lesion than fatty liver, is poorly defined. NASH is characterized by steatosis and inflammation, as well as hepatocyte ballooning degeneration or necrosis, and fibrosis. NASH has been reported worldwide, although geographic variations in prevalence are evident. In a recent study, NASH was documented in 26% of 81 non-alcoholic patients with marker-negative abnormal liver function tests. The prevalence of NASH in the general population has not been defined. In a large autopsy series of 351 non-alcoholic obese and non-obese patients, the prevalence of NASH was 6.3%. NASH has been described in obese adolescents as well as adults. Most cases occur in persons in the fourth to sixth decades of life. Women comprise 60-83% of patients with NASH in most clinical studies. Recent studies suggest however, that men may be afflicted equally.

Obesity is the condition most often reported in association with NASH. The earliest report of "fatty liver hepatitis," an early name for what was later called NASH, was in a cohort of obese patients. Obesity is described in 40 to 100% of patients with NASH, depending on the definition of obesity that is used. In a study of 100 morbidly obese patients undergoing gastric bypass surgery, 36% had some degree of steatohepatitis. Other studies have documented NASH in 9-26% of obese patients. The prevalence of NASH seems to correlate with the degree of obesity.

NAFLD has been associated with Type II diabetes mellitus and glucose intolerance, with or without superimposed obesity. Type II diabetes mellitus, hyperglycemia, or glucose intolerance has been described in 20 to 75% of adult patients with NASH. The association between type II diabetes mellitus and NASH is greatest in morbidly obese patients. The spectrum of NAFLD has been associated with insulin resistance and hyperinsulinemia even in lean subjects with normal glucose tolerance. The risk of NAFLD increases with the number of components of the metabolic syndrome X, including resistance, impaired glucose tolerance, hypertension, dyslipidemia, and visceral obesity conditions associated with with NAFLD are given in Tables 7 and 8.

Hyperlipidemia is found in a large proportion of patients with NASH. In published series, hypertriglyceridemia, hypercholesterolemia, or both were present in 18 to 20% of patients with NASH. Most patients with NASH have multiple risk factors, including obesity, type II diabetes mellitus, and/or hyperlipidemia [47, 52, 77].

TABLE 7
Conditions Associated with NAFLD

Acquired Metabolic Conditions: Obesity Diabetes mellitus Hyperlipidemia Rapid weight loss Total parenteral nutrition Acute starvation	**Inborn errors of Metabolism:** Wilson's Disease Abetalipoproteinemia Tyrosinemia Hypobetalipoproteinemia
Surgical Procedures: Jejuno-ileal bypass Biliopancreatic diversion Extensive small bowel resection Gastroplasty for morbid obesity	**Drugs/Toxins:** Amiodarone Glucocorticoids Perhexiline maleate Synethetic estrogens Tamoxifen 4,4' diethylaminoethoxyhexestrol (DHEAH) Isoniazid Industrial exposure to petrochemicals
Miscellaneous Factors: Partial lipodystrophy Jejunal diverticulosis with bacterial overgrowth	

The vast majority of patients with simple fatty liver are asymptomatic, and fatty liver is discovered as a result of an evaluation for associated medical conditions. Hepatomegaly may be present but stigmata of chronic liver disease are not seen. Liver functions test may be abnormal in up to 50% of patients, but are typically mild and do not correlate with the severity of steatosis.

Symptoms that have been described with NASH include vague right upper quadrant pain, fatigue, and malaise. Like fatty liver, NASH is often discovered incidentally during an evaluation for an unrelated medical condition. In contrast to simple fatty liver, most patients with NASH have elevated liver function tests and/or hepatomegaly. Hepatomegaly has been described in up to 75% of patients with NASH, although it is often difficult to detect on physical examination because of the body habitus. Stigmata of chronic liver disease are rare but may be seen in patients with NASH-associated cirrhosis. Laboratory features of NASH are nondiagnostic. Mild to moderate elevation of the serum aminotransferases are present in 70-100% of patients with NASH. There is no significant correlation between the degree of serum aminotransferase elevation and the histologic features. Serum levels of aspartate transaminase (AST) are characteristically higher than those of alanine transaminase (ALT), which contrasts with the pattern usually seen in alcoholic hepatitis. Alkaline phosphatase may be mildly elevated in approximately one-third of patients with NASH but bilirubin and albumin are usually normal. The prothrombin time (PT) was increased in 53% of patients in the study that first described NASH, but other studies have shown that prolongation of the PT is unusual. A small percentage of patients with NASH may have low-titer (≤ 1/320) antinuclear antibody (ANA) positivity. Antimitochondrial antibody (AMA), to hepatitis B surface antigen (HbsAg), and hepatitis C virus (HCV) serology are negative. Ceruloplasmin and α-lantitrypsin levels are within normal limits. Serum and hepatic iron stores may be elevated in patients with NASH but genetic hemochromatosis is relatively uncommon.

TABLE 8
Clinical and Laboratory Features of NASH

	Symptoms	***Signs***	***Laboratory Features***
Common	Asymptomatic (48-100%)	Hepatomegaly	2-4 fold elevation of ALT and AST AST/ALT < 1 in most cases Alkaline phosphatase slightly elevated in 1/3 Normal bilirubin, albumin, prothrombin time Elevated serum ferritin (53-62%)
Uncommon	Vague right upper quadrant pain Fatigue Malaise	Splenomegaly Spider angiomata Palmar erythema Ascites	Low titer (<1/320) ANA Elevated transferring saturation Cys282Tyr mutation of HFE gene

Hepatic steatosis develops in the setting of multiple clinical conditions and diseases including obesity, diabetes mellitus, alcohol abuse, protein malnutrition, total parenteral nutrition, acute starvation, corticosteroid therapy, and carbohydrate overload. In order to understand how steatosis develops, one has to first understand how the liver metabolizes lipids under normal conditions. In the fed state, dietary triglycerides are processed by the enterocyte into chylomicrons, which are secreted into the lymph. The chylomicrons are hydrolyzed into fatty acids by lipoprotein lipase located in the capillary endothelium. These free fatty acids are either transported to the liver, stored in adipose tissue as reesterified triglycerides, or used as energy sources by muscle. Free fatty acids are also supplied to the liver in the form of chylomicron remnants, which are then hydrolyzed by hepatic triglyceride lipase. During fasting, the fatty acids supplied to the liver are derived from hydrolysis of triglycerides stored in adipose tissue. This reaction is mediated by a hormone-sensitive lipase, which is stimulated by catecholamines, glucagons, and growth hormones, and inhibited by insulin. In the liver, the free fatty acids from all of these sources are either oxidized by mitochondria, used for triglyceride synthesis, or used to form phospholipids and cholesterol esters.

Hepatic triglyceride accumulation occurs when there is a shift in fatty acid metabolism to favor net lipogenesis rather than lipolysis. This can occur when the amount of fatty acid supplied to the liver from the intestine or adipose tissue exceeds the amount needed for mitochondrial oxidation, synthesis of phospholipids, and synthesis of cholesterol esters. This is the presumed mechanism for steatosis in the setting of obesity, diabetes mellitus, excessive dietary intake of fats and carbohydrates, acute starvation, and total parenteral nutrition (TPN). Triglycerides can also accumulate in the liver because of decreased synthesis of lipoproteins and decreased export of lipids from the liver. Decreased fatty acid oxidation with subsequent fatty infiltration of the liver may contribute to the genesis of steatosis, which is presumed to lead to the pathogenesis of NASH. Clinical and laboratory features of NASH are given in Table 8.

The exact stimulus that causes steatosis to progress to steatohepatitis and fibrosis in some patients is unclear [15, 16]. Lipid peroxidation and oxidative stress is emerging as the best candidate for the "second hit" in the pathogenesis of NASH. Recent studies suggest that hyperinsulinemia and insulin resistance may have a role in the pathogenesis of NASH even in patients without glucose intolerance. Insulin resistance and hyperinsulinemia, which are characteristic of IRS, may lead to steatosis because high levels of insulin block mitochondrial fatty acid oxidation, leading to accumulation of triglycerides of fatty acids in the liver. Increased concentration of intracellular fatty acids may be directly toxic to hepatocytes or lead to oxidative stress which leads to inflammation and fibrogenesis [21].

Bacterial endotoxin may also contribute to the development of NASH in some circumstances. Investigators at Johns Hopkins have recently demonstrated that genetically obese mice with severe steatosis have a much greater sensitivity to endotoxin than lean controls and rapidly develop NASH after exposure to low doses of bacterial lipopolysaccharide. The authors postulated that obesity promotes liver injury via a complex mechanism that involves Kupffer cell dysfunction, impaired phagocytosis, and chronic low-grade systemic endotoxemia, which then creates the environment where TNFα and other cytokines damage sensitized hepatocytes through lipid peroxidation.

Mitochondrial changes and altered hepatic energy homeostasis may also be important in the pathogenesis of NASH. Studies have shown that genetically obese mice and patients with NASH have severely impaired hepatic ATP homeostasis, with diminished capacity to recovery from hepatic ATP depletion, BMI correlated inversely with ATP recovery in NASH patients and controls [39].

It is unlikely that one of these mechanisms explains the pathogenesis of NASH in all affected patients. More likely, NASH develops as a consequence of a two-hit process, with the first hit being steatosis caused by a variety of mechanisms. After steatosis develops, a number of factors may incite the inflammatory response and fibrosis. The exact interplay between these factors remains to be elucidated and will be the source of exciting scientific investigation in the future.

Most patients with NAFLD are evaluated because of chronically elevated liver function tests, hepatomegaly, or both. The combination of history, physical examination, noninvasive blood tests, and radiologic examinations are useful for excluding other causes of liver disease. Laboratory testing should include a complete hepatic profile, CBC, PT, HCV antibody, HbsAg, iron indices, ceruloplasmin, ANA, α1-antitrypsin, and AMA. Hepatic ultrasound, the preferred imaging modality, reveals a "bright" liver of increased echogenicity. Ultrasound is 89-95% sensitive and 84-93% specific for steatosis, but only 57-77% sensitive and 85-95% specific for fibrosis. The diagnosis of NASH can be entertained only in the absence of significant alcohol use. The role of the liver biopsy in establishing the diagnosis of NASH has been debated. Many practitioners consider NASH a diagnosis of exclusion. One study showed that positive predictive value of the pre-biopsy diagnosis was only 56% for fatty liver. NASH is a histologic diagnosis and liver biopsy is the only diagnostic test that can reliably identify and quantify hepatic steatosis, inflammation, necrosis, and fibrosis. For these reasons, many hepatologists recommend that a liver biopsy be performed in all patients with persistently abnormal LFTs and fatty liver by ultrasound to distinguish simple fatty liver from NASH.

The optimal therapy for NAFLD has not been established in adults, weight loss has resulted in normalization of biochemical and ultrasonographic abnormalities in children with histologically-proven NASH, but this approach has not been examined in a controlled manner in adults. Several studies have reported improvement in liver chemistries and/or histology after weight loss in a small number of patients with NASH. Rapid weight loss has been associated with exacerbation of steatophepoatitis in morbidly obese patients; therefore weight loss should be moderate and monitored carefully [48, 49, 54, 99-102].

SLEEP APNEA

Sleep apnea is a serious, potentially life threatening condition that is far more common than generally understood. First described in 1965, sleep apnea is a breathing disorder characterized by brief interruption of breathing during sleep. It owes its name to a Greek word, apnea, meaning "want of breath." There are two types of sleep apnea: central and obstructive. Central sleep apnea, which is less common, occurs when the brain fails to send the appropriate signals to the breathing muscles to initiate respiration. Obstructive sleep apnea is far more common and occurs when air cannot flow into or out of the person's nose or mouth although efforts to breathe continue [33, 51].

In a given night, the number of involuntary breathing pauses or "apneic events" may be as high as 20 to 60 or more per hour. These breathing pauses are almost always accompanied by snoring between apnea episodes, although not everyone who snores has this condition. Sleep apnea can also be characterized by choking sensations. The frequent interruptions of deep, restorative sleep often leads to excessive daytime sleepiness and may be associated with an early morning headache.

Early recognition and treatment of sleep apnea is important because it may be associated with irregular heartbeat, high blood pressure, heart attack, and stroke.

Sleep apnea occurs in all age groups and both sexes but is more common in men (it may be under diagnosed in women) and possibly young African Americans. It has been estimated that as many as 18 million Americans have sleep apnea. Four percent of middle-aged men and 2 percent of middle-aged women have sleep apnea along with excessive daytime sleepiness. People most likely to have or develop sleep apnea include those who snore loudly and also are overweight, or have high blood pressure, or have some physical abnormality in the nose, throat, or other parts of the upper airway. Sleep apnea seems to run in some families, suggesting a possible genetic basis.

Certain mechanical and structural problems in the airway cause the interruptions in breathing during sleep. In some people, apnea occurs when the throat muscles and tongue relax during sleep and partially block the opening of the airway. When the muscles of the soft palate at the base of the tongue and the uvula (the small fleshy tissue hanging from the center of the back of the throat) relax and sag, the airway becomes blocked, making breathing labored and noisy and even stopping it altogether. Sleep apnea also can occur in obese people when an excess amount of tissue in the airway causes it to be narrowed. With a narrowed airway, the person continues his or her efforts to breathe, but air cannot easily flow into or out of the nose or mouth. Unknown to the person, this results in heavy snoring, periods of no breathing, and frequent arousals (causing abrupt changes from deep sleep to light sleep). Ingestion of alcohol and sleeping pills increases the frequency and duration of breathing pauses in people with sleep apnea.

Because of the serious disturbance in their normal sleep patterns, people with sleep apnea often feel very sleepy during the day and their concentration and daytime performance suffer. The consequences of sleep apnea range from annoying to life-threatening. They include symptoms suggesting depression, irritability, sexual dysfunction, learning and memory difficulties, and falling asleep while at work, on the phone, or driving. Untreated sleep apnea patients are 3 times (or more) likely to have automobile accidents [162], CPAP treatment reverses the increased risk. It has been estimated that up to 50 percent of sleep apnea patients have high blood pressure. It has recently been shown that sleep apnea contributes to high blood pressure. Risk for heart attack and stroke may also increase in those with sleep apnea [76].

a) **Obstructive Apnea**: Respiratory cessation occurs despite continued ventilatory effort indicating obstruction of the pharyngeal airway.

b) **Central Apnea**: Simultaneous cessation of all respiratory effort and airflow.

c) **Mixed Apnea**: Begins as a central event (no effort), but ultimately respiratory effort against an occluded pharyngeal airway begins.

d) **Hypopnea**: A 50% decrease in airflow lasting longer than 10 seconds associated with a 4% or greater fall in arterial oxygen saturation or arousal from sleep.

e) **Normal**: A normal individual will likely have less than 5 and certainly less than 10 disordered breathing events (apneas plus hypopneas) per hour of sleep. This is called the apnea-hypopnea index (AHI) or respiratory disturbance index (RDI).

PATHOPHYSIOLOGY OF OBSTRUCTIVE SLEEP APNEA

The adverse consequences of obstructive sleep apnea fall into three major categories: cognitive, quality of life, and cardiovascular. Each will be addressed briefly below.

a) **Cognitive**: This particular area will be addressed minimally as it has been well studied for a number of years. Patients with sleep apnea have disrupted sleep due to repetitive arousal. This leads to impaired vigilance with substantial somnolence during the day. This has been measured with both MSLT (Multiple Sleep Latency Test) and MWT (Maintenance of Wakefulness Test).

The patients also have impaired reaction time and decreased performance on a variety of neurocognitive tests.

The most glaring consequence of this cognitive dysfunction is the increased frequency of automobile crashes which occur 3-7 times more commonly in apnea patients than controls.

b) **Quality of Life**: Patients with sleep apnea have decreased quality of life on both general scales such as the SF-36 (Short Form Health Survey) and on disease specific scales. The SF-36 showed:

- Lower social functioning
- Limitation of function caused by physical and emotional reasons
- Lowered sense of well-being for mental health and energy.
- Poor adjustment.

Preliminary data suggest improvement in these Quality of Life scales with CPAP therapy.

c) **Cardiovascular**:

Hypertension (Systemic): There are currently very convincing data that sleep apnea contributes to the development of Systemic hypertension. These data take two forms.

- Human epidemiologic studies show at higher frequency of hypertension and a higher blood pressure (across the 24-hour day) in patients with sleep apnea when compared to controls. This was the case even after controlling for age, body mass index and gender.
- Animal studies in which tracheal obstruction was repetitiously produced at sleep onset in dogs have led to both nocturnal and durnal hypertension while acoustic arousal alone only led to nocturnally increased blood pressure.
- Arrhythmias: There is overwhelming data that apneas with oxygen desaturation lead to bradycardia. This can occasionally be extreme. The data supporting other arrhythmias are less convincing or consistent.

- Stroke: The relationship between apnea and stroke is controversial. Several studies have demonstrated an increased frequency of apnea in stroke patients shortly after the occurrence of the stroke. However, such studies do not prove a cause and effect relationship.
- Pulmonary Hypertension/cor pulmonale: A substantial amount of literature suggests that sleep apnea may lead to mild pulmonary hypertension when measured during wakefulness. However, if there are no other diseases besides apnea, the development of more severe pulmonary hypertension or cor pulmonale is quite rare. On the other hand, if there is walking hypoxemia (due to COPD, hypoventilation or other causes) in combination with sleep apnea, right ventribular dysfunction in association with important pulmonary hypertension may develop.
- Myocardial Infarction (MI): As with stroke, the data supporting a relationship between apnea and MI are incomplete. One study showed a substantially increased frequency of apnea in a group of patients having recently suffered MI when compared to a group without obvious coronary artery disease. Again, however, cause and effect was not demonstrated and we must await further data before firm conclusions can be reached.
- Death: There are a number of studies suggesting an increased mortality in patients with sleep apnea. Most such deaths appear to be cardiovascular in nature. However, due to methodological flaws in these studies, the impact of apnea on long-term survival is still poorly understood [33, 51, 55, 94].

TREATMENT OF OBSTRUCTIVE SLEEP APNEA

Simple Approaches: A variety of simple approaches have been used to treat sleep apnea over the years. These include:

1. Weight loss: If substantial weight is lost (diet or surgery) apnea commonly improves.
2. Maximize nasal patency: Poorly studied, but probably improves mild apnea.
3. Position control in bed: Avoiding the supine posture (uncomfortable object in the pajama shirt) will improve apnea in patients with positional apnea.

4. Avoid alcohol and sedatives near bedtime: Alcohol, in particular, has been shown to worsen apnea.

Nasal CPAP: Highly effective form of therapy. However, compliance is a major problem. The main problems patients have with CPAP include [94]:

1. Nasal drying/rhinorrhea: Treated with heated humidification, nasal steroids or nasal atrovent.
2. Mask discomfort: Many masks are currently available.
3. Difficulty breathing out against the pressure.
4. With careful attention to these problems, many believe compliance can be substantially improved.

Surgery: There are a variety of surgical approaches used to manage obstructive sleep apnea.

1. Uvulopalatopharyngoplasty (UPPP): This approach has been used for years and involves removing the uvula and varying portions of the soft palate. However, the success in reducing the AHI to >20 events/hour is about 40%.
2. Laser-assisted Uvuloplasty: Although this procedure is widely used in the treatment of snoring, the few studies assessing its efficacy in the treatment of apnea have been disappointing.
3. Mandibular procedures: There are two such procedures, the mandibular osteotomy with hyoid suspension and the mandibular-maxillary advancement. The former, often conducted in conjunction with UPPP, has about a 60-70% success rate. The advancement procedure is conducted in a limited number of centers, but in experienced ones, generally has a good outcome.
4. Radiofrequency Tissue Reduction: This is a new procedure for reduction in palatal size (may be applied to the base of the tongue as well). It is believed to reduce palatal size and decrease tissue compliance which will improve snoring and possibly treat sleep apnea. Only one study in humans has been published and it suggests that mild apnea (AHI<15) may improve.

DENTAL APPLIANCES

A variety of dental appliances have been used to treat sleep apnea. Most advanced the mandible opening of the airway behind the tongue. Their success is somewhat variable and often difficult to predict. However, they are often used in patients who do not tolerate CPAP.

Chapter 6

TREATMENT OF OBESITY

A. PATIENT READINESS ASSESSMENT

Loosing weight is a difficult process and a patient needs to be motivated. It is important to assess whether the patient really wants to lose weight and is motivated to do so. In addition, a readiness assessment should be made concerning psychological attitudes toward weight loss, ability to do physical activity, and ability to understand nutritional guidelines. It is also important to consider social support, family support, and family dynamics. Patient readiness assessment test is given in the Appendix. The influence of a physician has been shown to affect the patient's behavior toward weight loss. Discussion of diet and exercise and related health benefits with patients can sometimes motivate them to lose weight.

A comprehensive medical examination is important in determining how much weight a person should lose to achieve health benefits. Nutritional assessment form is included in the Appendix. The nutritional assessment should include:

1. Weight
2. Height
3. Waist measurement
4. Hip measurement
5. Waist/hip ratio (WHR)
6. BMI (given in the Appendix)
7. Medical problems
8. Over the counter medications
9. Supplements/herbs
10. Previous diets
11. Exercise habits
12. Family history of obesity
13. Behavioral evaluations
14. Weight-reduction
15. Readiness score

B. WEIGHT. The Ideal Body Weight (IBW) of the patient can be calculated in the following way:

Women IBW	**Men IBW**
100 lbs for 5 feet	106 lbs for 5 feet
5 lbs for additional inch	6 lbs for additional inch
e.g., 5′2″ = 100 + 10 = 110 lbs	e.g., 5′10″ = 106 + 60 = 166 lbs

Other considerations
Subtract 5 lbs for a very small framed person
Increase 5 lbs for medium frame
Increase 10 lbs for large frame

Ideal body weight has to be individualized for each patient. For example, for a 35-year old woman (medium frame) weighs 200 lbs, 5′2″. Her ideal body weight should be:

5′2″ = 100 + 10 + 5 + (medium frame) = 115 lbs

After interviewing the patient, you find that the patient has weighed about 145 lbs when she was 25 years old. She does not remember weighing less than that during her adult life. It will be very difficult for her to reach IBW of 115 lbs. The realistic goal of total weight loss should be set in consultation with the patient. Perhaps, in this case the realistic goal for this patient may be 140 lbs.

Height	Measurement of height is very important to assess BMI.
Waist Measurement	Waist circumference of ≥ 35 inches in women increases disease risk.
Hip Measurement	This measurement is important to determine WHR. WHR > .85 is associated with cardiovascular risk factor.
BMI	BMI values are given in the appendix. BMI provides the most clinically relevant measure of the person's weight status. BMI ≥ 25 indicates overweight and BMI ≥ 30 indicates obesity.

Medical Problems	Some of the medical problems may slow weight loss program. This should be taken into account when planning a diet program.
Medications	Some medications may increase hunger and the patient may feel hungry most of the time.
Behavioral Education	This should be part of the nutritional assessment. This will include patient's current eating practice, exercise habits, level of physical activity, previous dieting history, type of meals eaten, and frequency of eating out.

C. CALCULATION OF DAILY ENERGY REQUIREMENT

The daily energy requirements of an individual can only be estimated because measuring of the metabolic rate is impractical as it is time consuming and expensive. As a result, many physicians use equations developed by various research groups. The Basal Metabolic Rate (BMR) constitutes about 60% to 70% of the daily energy expenditure. Since the thyroid hormone regulates BMR, thyroid function tests are used in clinical practice to serve as indirect measures of BMR. This is important to know if the patient has hypothyroidism, which will indicate patient has low BMR.

Commonly used classic Harris-Benedict equations, involves measures of weight (kg), height (centimeters) and age. The equation is as follows.

Basal Energy Expenditure (BEE)

Women: BEE = 655 + [9.6 x weight (kg)]+(1.7 x height (cm) – (4.7 x age)

Men: BEE = 66+[13.7 x weight (kg)]+(5.6 x height (cm)–(6.8 x age)

This equation may not be practical to use everyday. The daily adult basal and physical activities can be calculated as follows:

I. Basal Energy Needs

A. Men: 1 Cal/kg/hr
B. Women: 0.9 Cal/kg/hr

Women's basal metabolic rate is 10% lower than men.

II. Activity Energy Needs

(VS) Very sedentary + 20%
(S) Sedentary + 30%
(MA) Moderately active + 40%
(VA) Very active + 50%

Example – Male (70 kg)

1. Basal energy needs

One Calorie x 70 kg x 24 hr = 1680 Calories

2. Activity

VS = 1680 + 336 = 2016
S = 1680 + 504 = 2184
MA = 1680 + 672 = 2352
VA = 1680 + 840 = 2520

Example – Female (60 kg)

1. Basal energy needs

0.9 Calorie x 60 kg x 24 hr = 1296

2. Activity

VS = 1296 + 259 = 1555
S = 1296 + 389 = 1685
MA = 1296 + 518 = 1814
VA = 1296 + 648 = 1944

D. DIET THERAPY

Calorie level is adjusted to meet individual's weight reduction goal. To lose about one pound per week, the patient needs to take 500 calories fewer than required calories. An average diet prescription for women is about 1200 calories per day for women and 1400 calories per day for men. For larger women and men, the prescription is about 1500 and 1800 calories respectively.

Nutrient Distribution

Nutrient distribution in the normal diet is recommended as follows:

1. **Proteins**. 20% of total Calories. Emphasis should be on fish, chicken, turkey, beans, and tofu.
2. **Fat**. Less than 30% of total Calories from fat. This part of the food composition plays very important part in weight reduction program.

3. **Carbohydrate**: 50% of total calories and this should come from complex carbohydrates and the diet should be high in fiber.

High fiber intake is important for good health and weight reduction. Dietary fiber is found only in plants: specifically plant foods, fruits and vegetables. There are two main types of fiber; insoluble and soluble (Table 1). Most fiber-containing foods have a mixture of both. Since the two fiber types help body in different ways, it's best to eat a variety of these foods.

TABLE 1
Insoluble and Soluble Fibers

Insoluble	Soluble
• Whole grains (wheat bran, whole grain breads and cereals) • Fruits and vegetables with edible skins and seeds (apples, pears, strawberries)	• Legumes (kidney beans, split peas) • Fruits and most vegetables • Oats and other grains

Why is Dietary Fiber Important?
Eating a diet with plenty of fiber-containing foods has both short- and long-term benefits. Short-term benefits are that fiber, particularly the insoluble type, can help prevent constipation and diverticulosis, a condition where the large intestine functions improperly. As a long-term benefit, it can help prevent some forms of cancer. Development of cancer depends on many factors. Eating a diet low in fat and high in grain products, fruits and vegetables that contain dietary fiber, may reduce risk for some types of cancer. Another bonus of a fiber-rich diet is that it tends to be low in fat, saturated fat and cholesterol.

How Much Dietary Fiber is needed?
Most Americans only get about half the 20 to 30 grams of fiber that is recommended per day. To boost daily fiber intake, one does not have to resort to using fiber supplements. Surprisingly, there are many easy and delicious ways one can get the fiber from everyday foods. In fact, it's better to obtain fiber from fiber-rich foods (e.g., whole grain breads, cereals, fruits and vegetables) since in addition to containing fiber, these foods also provide many other important nutrients.

How does one get More Fiber in the Diet?
There are lots of simple, natural ways to increase fiber intake. For example, fruits and vegetables with edible skins (like apples and

potatoes) should be eaten unpeeled, as the skin contains most of the fiber. Patients should be encouraged to eat 6 or more servings of bread, cereal, rice and pasta (concentrating on whole grain sources) and 5 or more servings of fruits and vegetables daily. The chart found on ***High Fiber Foods*** (Table 2), can help identify other great natural fiber sources.

Fiber intake should be gradually increased so that the digestive system has a chance to adjust. Plenty of fluids should be taken for proper digestion.

Fats

Dietary fats are composed chiefly of three fatty acids attached to a glycerol molecule. All fats are a combination of both saturated and unsaturated fatty acids. Fat is the most Calorically dense nutrient, supplying nine calories per gram. Therefore, a diet high in fat is generally high in calories. Reducing total fat intake and adhering to an exercise program can help an individual achieve weight loss.

Saturated Fats

Saturated fats are fatty acids with no double bonds. With the exception of palm, palm kernel, and coconut oils, saturated fats are solid at room temperature and come primarily from animal sources. Examples of foods high in saturated fat are butter, lard, beef and chicken fat, hot dogs, sausages, bacon, most cheeses, and whole milk. In the typical American diet, approximately 13 percent of the calories come from saturated fats. These fats contribute to atherogenesis by raising serum LDL cholesterol levels in animals and humans alike.

Unsaturated Fats

Unsaturated fats are classified as either polyunsaturated or mono-unsaturated. Fatty acids with one double bond are monounsaturated fats. Fatty acids with two or more double bonds are polyunsaturated fats. Both of these types of fats, found in fish and plant food sources, are generally liquid at room temperature.

Polyunsaturated Fats

The two major categories of polyunsaturated fats are omega-3 and omea-6 fatty acids. Vegetable oils such as corn, sunflower, safflower, and soybean contain omega-6 fatty acids. Polyunsaturated fats from these sources provide the essential omega-6 fatty acid. Linoleic acid is essential because it cannot be synthesized by the body and therefore, must be consumed in the diet. It is required by body to synthesize arachidonic acid, the precursor of prostaglandins. Essential fatty acid deficiency can result in dry, scaly dermatitis, increased susceptibility to infection, and impaired wound healing. Approximately 5 grams of linoleic acid per day (2 to 3 percent of total calories) are required to prevent essential fatty acid deficiency. Substituting foods rich in polyunsaturated fat for those high in saturated fat has been shown to decrease LDL cholesterol levels. Low-fat diets may also lower HDL levels in some individuals.

TABLE 2
High Fiber Foods

	Serving Size	**Grams of Fiber**
Bread, Cereal, Rice and Pasta		
Bran Muffin	1 muffin	5
Nabisco 100% Bran	1/3 cup	8
White Bread	1 slice	1
Whole Wheat Bread	1 slice	2
Oatmeal (cooked)	1 cup	4
Brown Rice (cooked)	¾ cup	3
White Rice (cooked)	¾ cup	1
Spaghetti (cooked)	1 cup	2
Popcorn	2-3/4 cups	3
Dry Beans, Nuts, and Seeds		
Baked Beans	½ cups	10
Kidney Beans	½ cups	8
Peanuts	3 tbsp	2
Cashews	¼ cup	1
Fruits		
Apples	1 medium	4
Banana	1 medium	1
Orange	1 medium	5
Orange Juice	8 fl ounces	0
Pear	1 medium	4
Prunes (dried)	5 prunes	3
Strawberries	8 medium	3
Vegetables		
Broccoli	3 spears	3
Carrots	½ cup	3
Corn	½ cup	2
Green Beans	2/3 cup	3
Potato (baked w/skin)	1 medium	3
Tomato (raw)	1 medium	1

Fish oils contain omega-4 fatty acids and have been shown to decrease blood pressure and triglyceride levels and increase clotting time. Recent research has also shown that individuals who consumed at least one meal per week of fatty fish rich in omega-3 fatty acids had a lower incidence compared to those who ate fatty fish less often. Because omega-3 fatty acids are concentrated in fish and shellfish, current recommendations are to advise to include these foods in the diet at least once a week. Fresh or canned tuna in water, salmon, sardines, and herring are good sources of omega-3 fatty acids. Patients with very high triglyceride levels may be prescribed fish oil supplements to produce a more rapid effect.

Monounsaturated Fats

Recently, monounsaturated fats have received attention because they do not raise LDL cholesterol levels. Canola and olive oils contain the highest percentage of monounsaturated fat. Oleic acid is the major fatty acid found in these oils. Epidemiological data suggest that people who live in certain Mediterranean countries such as Italy and Greece where olive oil is the basic cooking oil, have a lower incidence of heart disease. However the typical Mediterranean diet consists of considerably more fruits and vegetables and less meat than the typical American diet. Highly monounsaturated oils are especially good for cooking because they develop fewer free radicals when overheated than polyunsaturated oils.

Trans-Fatty Acids

Hydrogenation, the addition of hydrogen atoms to an unsaturated fat, changes the fat's structure, forming a trans-fatty acid. This process is often used by food manufacturers to give foods such as crackers, cookies, potato chips, and puddings a longer shelf life by making them less likely to turn rancid. Recent evidence suggests that trans-fatty acids may raise LDL cholesterol levels nearly as much as saturated fatty acids. There is no way to determine the amount of trans-fatty acids Americans consume. The newly revised food labels do not specify the amounts of trans-fatty acids in a product; the following current recommendations may be helpful to individuals who wish to decrease their intake of these substances:

1. Check ingredient labels on foods and limit intake of processed foods containing hydrogenated oils.

2. Limit intake of all fats. Use tub or squeeze margarines; the less solid the vegetable oil, the less hydrogenated fat it contains. Diet margarines are a better choice than regular margarine because

they contain more water, half the fat, and half the Calories.

3. Use liquid oil or a nonfat cooking spray on a nonstick pan for cooking.

4. Use olive oil or jelly as a spread on bread instead of butter or margarine.

Food Intake Guide

Food Exchange list can be used as a food guide. The exchange system of dietary management has been developed by the American Dietetic Association and the American Diabetes Association. It is based on the concept of nutritional equivalency. The foods are divided into six basic groups called the exchange lists. Each food item within a group contains about the same food value as other food items in that group, allowing exchange within groups, thus providing for variety in food choices or servings. The total number of exchanges per day depends on individual weight reduction plan. Exchange lists and Food Serving Guide are presented in Table 3

TABLE 3
Exchange – Calories

Food Group	**Calories per serving**						
		1200	1400	1500	1800	2000	2200
1. Fruit	60	2	3	4	5	5	6
2. Skim Milk	90	2	2	2	2	2	2
3. Bread	80	5	6	6	8	11	11
4. Meat	75	5	5	5	6	7	7
5. Vegetable	25	2	4	4	2	2	2
6. Fat	45	2	2	4	4	4	4

The above Table shows Food Groups, Calories per serving, number of servings needed in each diet. For example a person on 1200 Calorie Diet should take 2 servings/fruit, 2 serving of skim milk, 5 servings of bread, 5 servings of meat, 2 servings of vegetables and 2 servings of fat.

Food Serving Guide

Some people like to know how much to eat. The amount of food in each serving is given in Table 4.

TABLE 4
The Amount of Food in each Serving

Starch: Cereals, Grains, Pasta, Bread, Beans, Starchy Vegetables Guideline
One serving is: 1 slice bread – white, whole-wheat, pumpernickel, rye 1 small tortilla or waffle ½ English muffin, bagel, hot dog or hamburger bun, small pita bread ¾ oz pretzels ¾ cup unsweetened, dry cereal 1 cup broth-based soup 4-6 crackers 3 cups popcorn, popped, no fat added ½ cup cooked cereal, pasta, bulgur, or rice ½ cup cooked beans and peas (garbanzo, pinto, kidney, black-eyes) or corn ½ cup sweet potato or yam 1 small potato (3 oz) **Other Carbohydrates:** 1 tbs regular syrup, jam ¼ cup sherbet or sorbet 3 ginger snaps
Fruits
One serving is: 1 small fresh fruit ½ cup fruit juice ½ cup canned fruit 1 cup melon ¼ cup dried fruit 1 cup berries 17 small grapes
Milk and Yoghurt
90 calories: 1 cup nonfat or low-fat milk ¾ cup plain nonfat yogurt **120 calories:** 1 cup reduced-fat milk

¾ cup plain low-fat yogurt **150 calories:** 1 cup whole milk
Vegetables
One Serving is: 1 cup raw vegetables ½ cup cooked vegetables ½ cup tomato or vegetable juice Eat a different-colored vegetable – green, yellow, orange, red, white. There are many vegetables, including green beans, beets, broccoli, carrots, cauliflower, okra, peppers, spinach, tomatoes, and zucchini.
Protein
3 oz cooked chicken, turkey, fish, beef, pork, lamb, wild game is the size of a deck of cards 1 oz cheese is 1 slice ¼ cup cottage cheese or tuna is 1 oz ½ cup tofu is 1 oz 2 tablespoons peanut butter count as 1 oz 1 egg counts as 1 oz
Fats
1 teaspoon – margarine, butter, mayonnaise, oil 1 Tablespoon – reduced-fat margarine, reduced-fat mayonnaise, salad dressing, cream cheese, half-and-half cream 2 Tablespoons seeds – sesame, pumpkin, sunflower 2 Tablespoons – reduced-fat salad dressing, reduced-fat cream cheese, sour cream; chitterlings Other food high in fat are nuts, whole milk, cheese, high-fat meats like hot dogs, sausage, and bologna, snack foods, regular ice cream, fast foods, and fried foods.
Free Foods **These foods have less than 20 calories a serving. Enjoy! If a serving size is given, limit those foods to 3 a day**
1 tablespoon cream cheese, fat-free 1 tablespoon mayonnaise, fat-free 1 tablespoon salad dressing, fat-free ¼ cup salsa

2 servings of vegetables	
sugar-free gelatin	sugar-free gum
sugar substitutes	diet drinks
spices/herbs	mustard
lemon juice	nonfat cooking spray
water	hot pepper sauce

**These guidelines are developed by the "American Dietetic Association and American Diabetes Association".*

Nutritional Guidelines

Nutritional recommendations urge Americans to exercise an hour a day, boost their fiber intake and significantly cut back on fast foods.

Instead of setting a single average target for the maximum number of Calories people should consume every day – the previous guidelines advised about 2,900 calories a day for men and 2,200 calories for most women – these guidelines also conclude that how much people eat should be tied directly to how much physical activity they get. For example, a sedentary women might only need 1,800 calories a day, the report notes, but a very active woman the same age and size could eat up to another 1,000 calories a day to maintain a healthy body weight.

For the first time, the guidelines set a recommended daily intake for carbohydrates. Children and adults need a minimum of 130 grams a day of carbohydrates to provide enough glucose to the brain. That's about six times as much as what low-carbohydrate regimens like the Atkins diet advise during the weight-loss phase. Carbohydrates come from bread, crackers, pasta, fruit, vegetables, potatoes, beans and many other foods.

Issued by the National Academy of Sciences after more than two years of study, the report is called the Dietary Reference Intakes and takes the place of what were formerly called the Recommended Daily Allowances – better known as RDAs. This report is from the Academy revising all its dietary recommendations for the first time since 1989.

These guidelines also ease up a little on fat. Instead of urging a blanket approach that about 30 percent of total daily calories can come from fat, they say that a healthy diet can include from 20 percent calories from fat to as much as 35 percent, that upper limit echoes the latest guidelines issued by the National Heart, Lung and Blood Institute, but goes farther than current recommendations set by the American Heart Association.

Healthful fats are emphasized in these guidelines, which set a daily intake for two types of polyunsaturated fat that appear to help reduce sudden death from heart disease. These beneficial fats cannot be manufactured by the body and so need to be eaten every day. While dietary supplements can supply them, it is important to meet these requirements with food. Good sources include milk, nuts, avocados, olives, flaxseed, soybean as well as safflower, canola and corn oils.

The report prints the dangers of saturated fat such as that found in fatty cuts of meat or whole fat dairy products and of trans-fatty acids, which often appear in baked goods and fried foods. Dietary cholesterol, the report notes, should also be eaten sparingly because the body naturally makes all that it needs; all three of these fats help contribute to the risk of heart disease.

Fiber is a food that is often lacking in most people's diets. For this reason, the guidelines establish the first recommended dietary allowance for fiber, setting 38 grams for men ages 50 and younger and 25 grams a day for women the same ages, this requirement can be met by eating more fruit and vegetables, beans, and whole grains, such as whole wheat bread, oatmeal and other whole grain cereals and brown rice, the report notes.

Further revisions of these guidelines have been made.

Recommendations of the 2005 Dietary Guidelines by the Advisory Committee:

- Consume a variety of foods within and among the basic food groups while staying within energy needs
- Control calorie intake to manage body weight.
- Be physically active every day.
- Increase daily intake of fruits and vegetables, whole grains, and nonfat or low-fat milk and milk products.
- Choose fats wisely for good health.
- Choose carbohydrates wisely for good health.
- Choose and prepare foods with little salt.
- If you drink alcoholic beverages, do so in moderation.
- Keep food safe to eat.

This list makes a major departure form previous editions of *Dietary Guidelines for Americans* in that it does not include a message specifically directed toward sugars. This does not mean that the current Committee views the topic of sugars to be unimportant. On the contrary, the Committee provides a strong rationale for limiting one's intake of added sugars (that is, sugars and syrups that are added to foods during processing or preparation or at the table). The Committee's intent is to make this point clearly under new topic *"Choose Carbohydrates wisely for Good Health."*

Special nutrient recommendations are warranted for a few large subgroups of the population as follows:

- Adolescent female and women of childbearing age need extra iron and folic acid.
- Persons over age 50 benefit from taking vitamin B_{12} in its crystalline form from foods fortified with this vitamin or food supplements that contain vitamin B_{12}.
- The elderly, persons with dark skin, and persons exposed to little UV radiation may need extra vitamin D from vitamin D-fortified foods and/or supplements that contain vitamin D.

Control Calorie Intake to Manage Body Weight

Calorie intake and physical activity go hand in hand in controlling a person's weight. Calorie intake is emphasized under this message, physical activity under the next one.

To stem the obesity epidemic, most Americans need to reduce the amount of calories they consume. When it comes to weight control, calories do count—not the proportions of carbohydrate, fat, and protein in the diet. Energy expended must equal energy consumed to stay at the same weight. A deficit could be achieved by eating less, being more active physically, or combining the two. Since many adults gain weight slowly over time, even a small calorie deficit can help avoid weight gain. For example, a calorie deficit of 50 to 100 calories per day would enable many adults to maintain their weight rather than continuing to gain weight each year. for children who are gaining excess fat, a similar small decrease in energy intake can reduce the rate at which they gain weight so as they age they will grow into a healthy weight. Small changes maintained over time can make a big difference in body weight.

Monitoring weight regularly helps people know if they need to adjust their food intake or amount of physical activity to maintain their weight.

Limiting the portion sizes that a person takes or serves to others often helps reduce calorie intake, especially if the food is high in energy density. On the other hand, consuming large portions of raw vegetables or low-fat soups may help limit one's intake of other foods that are more energy dense. The healthiest way to reduce calorie intake is to reduce one's intake of added sugars, solid fats, and alcohol—they all provide calories, but they do not provide essential nutrients.

Be Physically Active Every Day

Making moderate physical activity a part of an adult's daily routine for at least 30 minutes per day promotes fitness and reduces the risk of chronic health conditions such as obesity, hypertension, diabetes, and coronary artery disease. (Walking at a brisk pace [3 to 4 miles per hour] is an example of a moderate physical activity.) Moderate physical activity for an hour each day can increase energy expenditure by about 150 to 200 calories, depending on body size. If not offset by increased calorie intake, this increase in physical activity could be helpful in preventing weight gain. Many adults need to participate in up to 60 minutes of moderate to vigorous physical activity on most days to prevent unhealthy weight gain, while adults who have previously lost weight may need 60 to 90 minutes of moderate physical activity daily to help avoid regain of weight. Children and adolescents need at least 60 minutes of moderate to vigorous physical activity on most days for the maintenance of good health and fitness and for healthy weight gain during growth. Compared with moderate physical activity, vigorous physical activity provides greater benefits for physical fitness and burns more calories per unit time.

Sources: *2005 Report of the Dietary Guidelines Advisory Committee (every 5 years an Expert Dietary Guidelines Advisory Committee is appointed to make recommendations to the Secretaries of HHS, USDA, concerning revisions of Dietary Guidelines for Americans).*

PYRAMIDS

USDA's Food Group Pyramid can also be used as a weight reduction guide as shown in Figures 1 and 2.

Numbers correspond to exchanges given in Table 3. Serving Sizes are given in Table 4 Serving Guide.

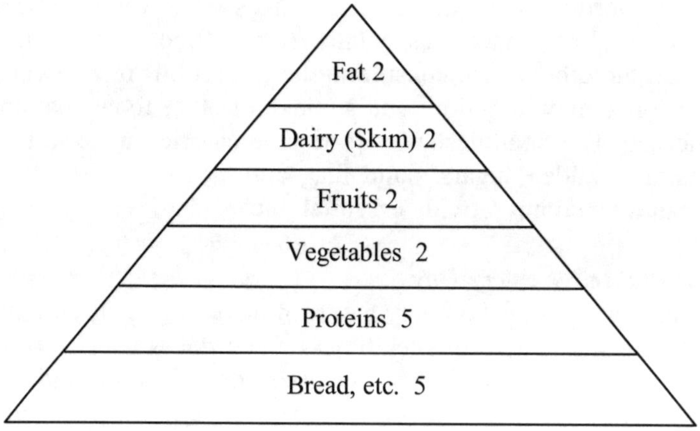

FIGURE 1
Weight Reduction Pyramid (For women 1200 Calories)

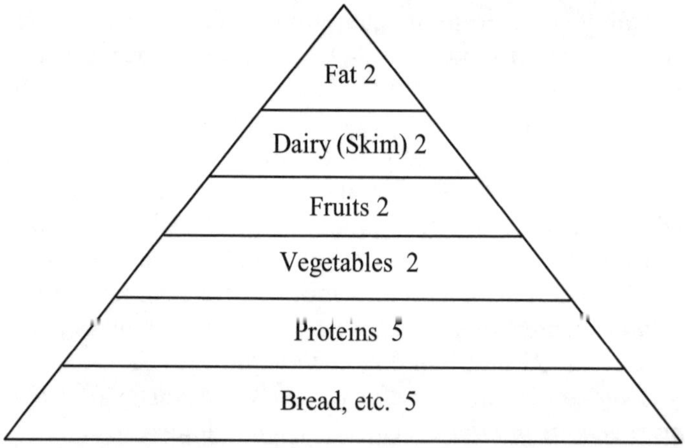

FIGURE 2
Weight Reduction Pyramid (For men 1400 Calories)

E. PRINCIPLES OF BEHAVIORAL TREATMENT

The goal of behavioral treatment is to help obese patients identify and modify eating, activity, and thinking habits that contribute to their excess weight. This approach recognizes that body weight is affected by factors other than behavior. These factors include genetic, metabolic, and hormonal influences that likely predispose some persons to obesity and may set the range of possible weights that an individual can achieve. While recognizing that biology may set a range of possible weights, behavioral therapy helps obese individuals develop a set of skills (e.g., a low-fat diet, a high activity lifestyle, a realistic plan) to regulate weight at the lower end of that range, even though patients may remain overweight after treatment [22, 26, 80, 149, 164].

Behaviors are often prompted by antecedent or simultaneous events, which, if repeated, become strongly linked. For example, eating may be triggered by negative emotions, long periods of dietary restriction, watching a favorite TV show, or socializing with friends. The more often two things are paired together, the stronger the connection between the two so that eventually, the presence of one triggers the other. For example, after repeatedly eating ice cream while watching a favorite TV show, just seeing a commercial for the favorite show may trigger a craving for ice cream. Behavioral treatment, as described subsequently, attempts to identify and disconnect the triggers and overeating. Although eating can be triggered by one factor, it is more typical that a number of factors lead to overeating.

Behavioral treatment has several distinguishing features. First, it is goal-directed. It specifies clear goals in terms that can be easily measured. A specific goal can be walking three times per week, lengthening meal duration by 10 minutes.

Treatment is process oriented. It is more than helping people to decide what they want to accomplish; it is helping them to find how to do so. Once a goal is specified, patients are encouraged to examine factors that help or hinder goal achievement. In cases for which behavior is not implemented, attention is devoted to finding new strategies or to removing roadblocks. This skill-building philosophy conceptualizes weight management as a set of skills to be learned rather than as will power.

Behavioral approaches advocate small rather than large changes. This approach is based on the learning principle of successive approximation, in which incremental steps are taken to achieve more distant goals. Making small changes gives patients successful experiences on which to build, rather than attempting drastic changes, which are typically short-lived.

Behavioral treatment usually includes multiple components, such as self-monitoring, nutrition, stimulus control, slowing eating, exercise, problem solving, and cognitive restructuring. These components comprise the behavioral package, which has been summarized in self-help manuals such as the Learn Program for Weight Control. Three components of behavioral treatment are self-monitoring, exercise, and cognitive restructuring.

F. SELF-MONITORING

Self-monitoring is the most important of behavioral treatment. Although self-monitoring is used for eating, exercise, and thinking patterns, the focus here is on the self-monitoring of food intake. Several studies have shown that self-monitoring of intake correlates with successful long-term weight control. Initially, patients are instructed to keep daily records of their food intake (without attempting to change their diet), including the type, amount, and Caloric content. Patients then reduce their calorie intake by approximately 500 to 700 kcal per day to achieve a weight loss of approximately one pound per week. Over time, patients' record information about times, places, and feelings associated with eating. Such records are critical because they provide the information necessary to identify the various components of the behavior chain. Record keeping also serves to decrease, although not eliminate, the tendency of lean and obese persons to underestimate their food intake.

The behavioral approach to physical activity is that any activity is better than none. Rather than worrying about reaching some activity threshold (e.g., 30 minutes at 80% of maximum heart rate), efforts are directed toward increasing activity along a continuum. This goal can be accomplished by increasing programmed or lifestyle activity. Programmed activity typically consists of aerobic exercise (e.g., walking, biking, or swimming), engaged in for a set period of time (i.e., 20 to 40 minutes) at a relatively high-intensity level (i.e., 60% to 80% of maximum heart rate) that is planned ahead of time. Lifestyle activity involves becoming more active during the course of one's daily routine, as follows:

Take the stairs
Stand while on the telephone
Put away the remote control
Get off the bus a stop early
Choose active vacations
Avoid using children to fetch things
Take the long way around
Choose outdoor activities
Make several trips up the stairs

Answer the phone in another room
Hand-deliver messages
Park further away from entrances
Use a bathroom further away
Go out for entertainment (i.e., museums, fairs)
Move during commercials

G. COGNITIVE RESTRUCTURING

Cognitive restructuring teaches patients to identify, challenge, and correct the irrational thoughts that frequently undermine weight control efforts. These thoughts tend to occur in two principal areas: dealing with setbacks and accepting less-than-desired weight losses. Cognitive techniques are particularly helpful in dealing with lapse or setback situations. The interventions focus on accurately identifying the setback for what it is – a temporary lapse from which it is possible to recover. Once the event has been realistically assessed; efforts are directed at examining how the lapse occurred and how it can be prevented in the future.

H. BEHAVIOR MODIFICATION

Behavior modification is important in the treatment of obesity. Changing behavior is the only way to change a patient's weight permanently. Behavior modification focuses on gradual, permanent changes in eating and exercise habits. There are six ways of altering behavior that will help in maintaining weight loss: educating about nutrition, changing eating habits, increasing physical activity, altering attitudes, developing support systems, and changing unrealistic goals and false beliefs about weight loss

A summary of controlled trials with behavior therapy and low Calorie diet shows increasingly improving results over the past 30 years. This is related to more intense and longer treatment periods and prolonged maintenance follow-up. If maintenance is not taken seriously, weight regain tends to be the rule. Because of the longer treatment periods, attrition has decreased. If weight maintenance is to be sustained, prolonged follow-up must be done.

Behavior modification, with a focus on self-control, a gradual and permanent change in habits, an educational approach toward the patient by the physician, and incorporation of an individual's food preferences into dietary planning, is pivotal to successful weight loss. The physician must not demand perfection and should understand that there will be slips along the way [149, 164].

Some of the other tips that may be considered by the physician:

1. **Setting Goals**. The patient must be an active participant in setting goals for losing by behavior modification. It is important for the physician to emphasize that the patient should keep the appointment even if the goals have not been met. Setting goals should be a collaborative effort. Once goals are selected, an action plan can be devised to implement change. Goals must be attainable. Patients should be encouraged to select short-term goals. If a previous goal was missed by a wide margin, it may be useful to lower the goal.
2. **Recording diet and exercise patterns in a dairy**. Self-monitoring of a behavior usually changes the behavior in the desired direction. Suggested format of the diary is given in the appendix. Regular self-monitoring of weight is also important. The frequency of weighing must be established after discussion with the patient. In some instances, patients can drop by for a weight check.
3. **Avoid a chain reaction**. Separate the association of eating from the cue. Patients should not eat while watching television. Other helpful behavior modification tips include:

    - Eating slowly
    - Eating lots of vegetables
    - Using smaller portions

Behavior modification list is given in the appendix.

I. SHORT-TERM PSYCHOLOGICAL BENEFITS OF WEIGHT LOSS

Conventional weight loss treatments combining dietary control with increased exercise and other lifestyle changes are reliably effective in producing short-term weight loss in mild to moderate obesity. Studies using objective measures have consistently shown beneficial effects of treatment-induced weight loss on negative effects (anxiety and depression), self-esteem, and body image.

More conventional, self-initiated dieting also is associated with adverse psychological effects in normal weight young women. Cross-sectional studies of adolescent girls have indicated that independent of the effect of body weight itself, dieting is correlated with feelings of failure, lowered self-esteem, and social anxiety. Prospective research has shown that dieting predicts stress rather than vice versa.

Several lines of evidence suggest that dieting is closely linked to disordered eating and bulimia nervosa in women. Clinical descriptions consistently indicate that patients with bulimia nervosa almost always report that their binge-eating began when they were on a diet. Dieting is often neglected feature of bulimia nervosa and one of the most difficult to change.

Eating disorders are most common in the specific populations that are most invested in dieting and weight loss – predominantly white, middle- to upper-class females. There is an overall correlation between cultural pressure to be thin and prevalence of eating disorders both across and within different ethnic groups. A prospective study of 1,010 high school girls in London showed that compared with nondieters, dieters were significantly more likely to develop an eating disorder one year later.

Studies have shown that restrained eaters differ from nondieters or unrestrained eaters in the amount of food they eat after having consumed an actual or perceived high-calorie preload. In these studies, unrestrained eaters typically regulate their eating so that following a preload; they eat less in a subsequent taste-test than those who do not receive a preload. Restrained eaters typically regulate their intake in the absence of a preload but eat significantly more in a taste-test following consumption of a preload versus no preload, or they simply fail to regulate, that is, decrease their consumption. This pattern of disinhibited eating has been termed counterregulation and has been put forward as an experimental analog of binge-eating.

Dieting may not be as closely linked to binge-eating in obese patients as in normal weight bulimia nervosa. Research has shown that only a minority of obese binge-eaters reported being on a strict diet at the time binge-eating began and that obese binge eaters engage in less dietary restraint than normal weight patients with bulimia nervosa.

Although dieting is associated with the onset of eating disorders, the precise nature of this relationship remains to be established. Some investigators consider dieting to be a necessary but not sufficient cause of eating disorders, whereas others see it only as an antecedent.

In linking dieting to the development of disordered eating and eating disorders, it is important to note that there are different types of dieting and dieters. Dieters may vary both in the pattern and content of daily eating behavior. It can be hypothesized that the more chaotic the everyday eating behavior, the higher the risk of developing bulimia.

Whether dieting is a necessary condition or simply an antecedent of binge-eating, it cannot be a sufficient casual condition. The majority of adolescent and young adult women in the United States are typically on one form of diet or another. Yet only a small fraction of the women who diet develop an eating disorder. Some other factor or set of factors must interact with dieting-induced mechanisms to cause eating disorders. These risk factors may range from genetic predisposition and biological vulnerability through personality and individual psychopathology to familial influence.

J. MECHANISM WHEREBY DIETING LEADS TO BINGE-EATING

Dieting has a variety of biological, cognitive, and affective consequences that may predispose to binge-eating. At the cognitive level, unrealistically rigid standards of dietary restraint, coupled with a sense of deprivation, may leave the dieter vulnerable to loss of control over eating following perceived or actual transgression of the diet. The mere perception that they have eaten a high-calorie, forbidden food (regardless of actual caloric content) suffices to trigger counterregulation in restrained eaters in laboratory studies. Beyond its psychological effects of frustration and deprivation, dieting can be associated with different conditioning processes that may predispose to binge-eating. First, it may increase the appeal of forbidden or binge foods (typically those high in fat and sugar) directly by nutritional preference conditioning. Second, terminating meals because of a self-imposed limit rather than satiation, combined with variability in intake (skipping meals), can extinguish conditioned satiety responses and condition increasingly larger meal sizes.

Dieting may cause stress or make the dieter more vulnerable to its effects. To the extent that stress is a precipitant of binge eating, as bulimic patients report, this is another indirect means by which dieting may contribute to disordered eating.

K. FUTURE RESEARCH DIRECTIONS

Implications for Obesity Treatment

The short-term effects of weight loss cannot be considered apart from the consistent finding that this reduction is not maintained in the long term. For the majority of obese individuals, weight loss inevitably means weight regain. For most patients, this involves a recurring cycle of success and failure. Whereas the biological consequences of weight cycling have been studied in some detail, the psychological impact has been neglected. Critics of dietary treatments of obesity assert that the impact is typically devastating, sabotaging self-esteem and adding to the existing social stigma of obesity, the validity of these claims must be decided on the basis of systematic research rather than anecdotal observations. The treatment of obesity has not avoided the patient's uniformity myth. Patients typically receive the same highly standardized program. Some may be more vulnerable to adverse effects of a particular dietary treatment than others.

L. EXERCISE

Over 66% of American adults do not exercise on a regular basis, and many do not exercise at all. The technological revolution means that we have energy-saving instruments for just about everything, including the car, dishwasher and vacuum cleaner. In addition, we have replaced recreational activities with watching television. Television viewing contributes greatly to inactivity and is correlated with obesity. We are eating more than ever before, and we are less and less active, so that our expenditure does not keep up with our intake 6, 34, 53, 105, 130].

To remain weight stable, energy expenditure must equal food intake. If energy expenditure is less than food intake, weight gain will occur.

Exercise Improves Overall Fitness:

- Improves cardiovascular function
- Lowers LDL levels
- Increases HDL cholesterol levels
- Lowers blood pressure
- Improves glucose tolerance
- Lowers mortality rate

There are two types of activities. The first includes the routine daily activities that are integral to a person's life, such as walking, activities associated with one's occupation, and activities associated with maintenance of the house, the yard, etc. Much can be done to increase the energy expenditure of this component. Examples are walking rather than riding to the train station for commuting, getting off the bus at an earlier stop and walking a few blocks to work, walking up and down stairs rather than taking elevators, pushing a lawnmower rather than riding, and walking a dog twice a day. The second type consists of more structured exercise activities. These can range from simple walking to jogging, aerobics, swimming, tennis, golf and team sports. Generally, aerobic sports are preferred over resistance training, because there is a positive effect not only on weight but also on cardiovascular fitness. However, some resistance training will tend to build up lean body mass (muscle) and decrease fat and is, therefore, important. Physical inactivity is more prevalent in:

- Women than men
- African Americans, and Hispanics than whites
- Elderly than younger
- Less affluent than more affluent

The most popular physical activities in adults are walking, gardening and yard work. Fifty percent of American youths aged 12-21 years are not vigorously active on a regular basis. Enrollment in daily physical education classes declined by half of high school students between 1991 and 1995. Exercise declines dramatically during adolescence.

Exercise in health and disease

Overall mortality:

- High levels of regular exercise are associated with low mortality for both older and younger adults.
- Those who are moderately active on a regular basis have lower mortality rates than those who are least active.

Cardiovascular disease:

- Regular exercise or cardiorespiratory fitness decreases the risk of cardiovascular disease mortality in general and of coronary artery disease mortality in particular.
- Existing data are not conclusive regarding the relationship between exercise and stroke.

- The level of decreased risk of coronary heart disease associated with regular exercise is similar to that of other lifestyle factors such as avoidance of cigarette smoking.
- Regular exercise prevents or delays the development of high blood pressure. Exercise reduces blood pressure in people with hypertension.

Cancer:

- Regular exercise is associated with a decreased risk of colon cancer.
- There is no association between exercise and rectal cancer. Data are inconclusive regarding a relationship between exercise and endometrial, ovarian and testicular cancer.
- Data are inconsistent despite extensive studies regarding the association between exercise and breast or prostate cancer.

Non-insulin dependent diabetes:

- Regular exercise lowers the risk of developing non-insulin dependent diabetes.
- A patient with type 2 diabetes who starts a regular exercise activity program is likely to derive benefit in terms of glycemic control and other health variables.

Osteoarthritis:

- Regular exercise is important for maintaining normal muscle strength, joint function and joint structure. The range of exercise recommended is not associated with joint damage or development of osteoarthritis. The levels of exercise recommended may be beneficial for individuals with arthritis.
- Competitive athletics may be associated with osteoarthritis in a later life, but this is more likely to be related to sport injuries.
- Once a quantitative threshold for high levels of exercise is exceeded, the risk of musculoskeletal injuries increases.

Osteoporosis:

- Weight bearing exercise is important for normal skeletal development during childhood and adolescence and for achieving and maintaining peak bone mass in young adults.
- In the absence of estrogen replacement therapy it is unclear whether resistance or endurance of exercise can reduce the accelerated rate of bone loss in postmenopausal women.

Overall analysis of the studies suggest that regular exercise is likely to be a benefit in preventing accelerated bone loss in postmenopausal women. Overall analysis of the studies suggest that regular exercise is likely to be a benefit in preventing accelerated bone loss in postmenopausal women.

Risk of Falling:

- There is promising evidence that strength training and other forms of exercise in older individuals preserves the ability to maintain independent living and reduce the risk of falling.

Obesity:

- Lower levels of activity related both to exercise and non-exercise activity results in fewer calories being expended and consumed. This contributes to the prevalence of obesity in the United States.
- Exercise may favorably affect body fat distribution.

Mental Health:

- Exercise appears to relieve symptoms of depression and anxiety and improve mood.
- Regular exercise may reduce the risk of developing depression, although further research is needed on this topic.

Health related Quality of Life:

- Exercise appears to improve health related quality of life by enhancing psychological well-being and improving physical functioning in persons compromised by poor health.

Physiological responses to Long-term Adaptations to Exercise:

- People of all ages and of both genders undergo physiological adaptation to exercise.
- Exercise has numerous physiological benefits. Most widely noted are the effects on cardiovascular and musculoskeletal systems but there are also proven benefits on metabolic, endocrine, and immune system.
- Most of the demonstrated physiological benefits of exercise training diminish within two weeks if exercise is substantially reduced or stopped. Effects disappear within 2-8 months after exercise is discontinued.

Interventions:

- Little is understood regarding how to initiate and promote exercise. Some interventions have been successful at promoting exercise in schools, work sites and healthcare settings.
- Determination of the most effective and cost effective intervention for successfully achieving exercise interventions is yet to be determined.
- Influences on physical activity include:

1. Confidence in ones ability to engage in physical activity (self-efficacy)
2. Enjoyment of physical activity
3. Support from others
4. Positive beliefs concerning the benefits of physical activity
5. Lack of perceived barriers to being physically active
6. Potential impact of interventions based on individuals aged 6-16 years has received emphasis from statutory bodies.
7. Emphasis is being placed on preventing a fall-off of activity that occurs sharply with adolescents.
8. School-based interventions have been shown to be successful in increasing exercise levels.
9. Individual understanding, work schedules and health limitations are critical for success. Accumulating exercise over the course of the day has been included in recent recommendations from CDC and ACFM and NIH as well as the Surgeon General.
10. Most individuals who embark on strenuous exercise programs do not sustain their participation.
11. Exercise that occurs in several short sessions has been shown to have similar cardiorespiratory fitness compared to exercise that occurs in one longer session such as 30 minutes. Health benefits of intermittent activity such as this have yet to be comprehensively demonstrated.
12. Lifetime physical activities that can be enjoyed throughout life should be emphasized.
13. Special efforts are required to meet the needs of special populations such as those individuals with disability, racial and ethnic minorities, people with low income and the elderly. Investigation into successful interventions in these groups is necessary. Understanding diverse popu-

lations will make it simpler to provide recommendations for intervention.

Health Problems Associated with Exercise:

- Health problems are associated with exercise, particularly in excess, particularly musculoskeletal injury.
- Most musculoskeletal injuries related to exercise are believed to be preventable by gradually working up to a desired level of activity and by avoiding excessive amounts of activity.
- Serious cardiovascular events can occur with physical exertion, but the net effect of regular exercise is of benefit.
- There are serious associated health problems such as myocardial infarction and sudden death that occur primarily among sedentary people with advanced atherosclerotic disease who engage in strenuous activity to which they are unaccustomed. Sedentary people, particular those with pre-existing health conditions, who wish to increase their exercise should, therefore, gradually build up to the desired level of exercise. Even in people who are regularly active, the risk of myocardial infarction or sudden death is somewhat increased during physical exertion, but their overall risk of these outcomes is lower than for people who are sedentary.

Conclusions and Recommendations:

Exercise reduces the risk of:

- Premature overall mortality
- Premature coronary artery disease
- Hypertension
- Colon cancer (most likely)
- Diabetes mellitus
- Exercise improves mental health
- Exercise is likely to be important for sustenance of muscles, bones and joints.
- People of all ages irrespective of gender benefit from regular exercise.
- There are significant health benefits to be obtained from moderate amounts of exercise when performed on most, if not all, days of the week. Examples would include 30 minutes of brisk walking or leaf raking per day, 15 minutes of running per day, or 45 minutes of playing volleyball.

- Through a modest increase in daily activity most Americans can improve their health and quality of life.
- People of all ages should include a minimum of 30 minutes of exercise of moderate intensity such as brisk walking on most, if not all, days of the week.
- Cardiorespiratory endurance activity should be supplemented with strength developing exercises at least twice a week to improve musculoskeletal health and maintain independence in performing the activities of daily life as well as reduce the risk of falling.
- People with chronic disease such as cardiovascular disease and diabetes mellitus or those who are at risk of disease such as these should consult a physician before beginning a new exercise program. Men over the age of 40 and women over the age of 50 should consult with a physician before they begin vigorous exercise activity.
- Previously sedentary individuals should embark on exercise programs that start with short durations of moderate intensity activity and gradually increase the duration or intensity until the goal is reached.
- Individuals who can maintain a regular regimen of activity that is of longer duration or of more vigorous intensity, are likely to derive greater benefit. For example, 60 minutes of brisk walking is likely to derive greater health benefits than 30 minutes of walking.
- Promote physical activity through:

    1. Promoting self-efficacy
    2. Promoting the enjoyment of physical activity
    3. Promoting support for physical activity
    4. Promoting positive beliefs concerning the benefits of physical activity
    5. Eliminating/diminishing barriers to being physically active

Source: *Physical Activity and Health, a report of the Surgeon General, US Dept of Health and Human Services 1996, www.cdc.gov/nccdphp/sgr/summary.htm*

M. DRUG THERAPY

Criterion for Initiating Drug Therapy

- BMI > 30 or waist circumference > 40 inches for males or 35 inches for females, or BMI > 27 with obesity risk factor should be present before drug therapy for weight loss is considered.

- Medication therapy for obesity is appropriate only as an adjunct to a regimen of diet, exercise, and behavioral modification.
- Concurrent use of noradrenergic and serotonergic obesity medications is contraindicated in the presence of monoamine oxidase inhibitors, and extreme caution is needed with other serotonergic combinations.
- Exposure to some appetite suppressants (fenfluramine derivatives) can result in cardiac valve disease. Valvular insufficiency may improve after stopping exposure to drug.
- Obese individuals with concurrent diseases such as diabetes and hypertension require intensive monitoring when undertaking a weight loss program.
- Some herbal and food supplement diet agents contain sources of pharmacologically active substances that should be used with caution or avoided in obese patients with conditions such as diabetes, hypertension, and significant cardiovascular disease.
- The FDA does not regulate labeling of herbal and food supplement diet agents and content is not guaranteed.
- There is a high probability of weight regain when obesity pharmacotherapy is discontinued [29, 32, 87, 148, 174].

NORADRENERGIC AGENTS

Phentermine

Phentermine is structurally similar to amphetamine but it has less severe central nervous system stimulation and a lower abuse potential. Its mechanism of action is related to enhanced norepinephrine and dopamine neurotransmission. Phentermine is available in both immediate-release and sustained-release formulations. However, the value of sustained-release formulations can be questioned based upon the reported phentermine plasma half-life of 12 to 24 hours. A single dose of 30 mg once daily in the morning provides effective appetite suppression throughout the day. Divided doses of 8 mg immediately prior to meals, however, are common. Doses above 30 mg daily do not improve effectiveness. Evening or nighttime dosing should be avoided because of insomnia. Significant increases in blood pressure, palpitations, and arrhythrmias can occur with phentermine administration. Use is not advisable in hypertensive patients and those with unstable cardiovascular function. The potential for hypertensive crisis with coadministration of phentermine and monoamine oxidase (MAO) inhibitors is noted in product labeling because of the documented cases of this syndrome seen with coadministration of amphetamine or noradrenergic derivatives and MAO inhibitors. Similar warnings have been noted regarding concomitant use of tricyclic antidepressants, but this is less well documented. With MAO inhibitors, a minimum washout time of 14 days prior to use of any adrenergic agent is suggested to avoid excessive adrenergic stimulation syndromes. Phentermine use is contraindicated in patients who are abusers of substances such as cocaine, phencyclidine, and methamphetamine, again because of the potential for excessive adrenergic stimulation syndromes and abuse potential. Mydriasis from adrenergic stimulation can worsen glaucoma, and patients diagnosed with glaucoma should not receive phentermine. Diabetic patients may experience altered insulin or oral hypoglycemic dosage requirements soon after beginning therapy and prior to any substantial weight loss.

Phentermine is an effective adjunct to diet, exercise, and behavior modification for producing weight loss in excess of that seen with placebo. Intermittent phentermine therapy appears to elicit comparable weight loss when compared to continuous use. However, most individuals experience weight regains, during therapy and generally always after discontinuing use. In spite of its extensive off-label use in combination with the fenfluramine derivatives and the occurrence of cardiac valvulopathy, phentermine currently remains on the market as a short-term pharmacotherapy for obesity.

Mazindol

Although chemically distinct from amphetamines and phentermine, Mazindol's tricyclic structure results in amphetamine-like appetite suppression. Direct stimulation of hypothalamic activity and norepinephrine reuptake inhibition are potential Mazindol mechanisms. Mazindol undergoes extensive hepatic metabolism, and approximately 50% of an administered dose is recovered in urine, mostly as conjugated metabolites. The pharmacokinetics of Mazindol has not been extensively described; however, dosing is based upon an elimination half-life of 10 hours. Clinically, the drug is given once daily, 1 to 3 mg, prior to the morning or noon meal. However, some clinicians employ multiple small doses, 1 mg, given just prior to meals. Efficacy trials of single versus multiple daily doses are not available. Dry mouth commonly occurs with Mazindol use and difficulty with urination is possible. Mazindol use results in fewer Central Nervous System stimulant complaints than either phentermine or the amphetamines. Additionally, fewer cardiovascular adverse effects have been reported, and thus obese patients with mild to moderate hypertension may be treated with Mazindol. Contraindications for use are similar to phentermine and include concurrent MAO inhibitors, glaucoma, symptomatic cardiovascular disease, and stimulant substance abuse. Mazindol has been noted to cause lithium toxicity with concurrent use. Early studies in type II diabetic patients treated with Mazindol demonstrated no need for changes in oral hypoglycemic therapy. More recently, improved insulin sensitivity with Mazindol treatment was documented using euglycemic clamp studies. Caution and close monitoring of insulin or oral hypoglycemic dosage needs are advisable when treating obese diabetic patients with this therapy. Several placebo-controlled trials have demonstrated the effectiveness of Mazindol as a short-term therapy for weight reduction.

Diethylpropion

Diethylpropion stimulates norepinephrine release from presynaptic storage granules. Increased adrenergic neurotransmitter concentrations activate hypothalamic centers, which results in decreased appetite and food intake. This drug undergoes extensive first-pass hepatic metabolism. Active metabolites are renally eliminated and account for approximately 70% of administered dose. The elimination half-life of these metabolites is approximately 8 hours. Less than 10% of the parent compound is recovered in urine. No specific dosing recommendations exist for use in patients with renal or hepatic insufficiency. Diethylpropion can be taken in divided daily doses, generally 25 mg three times daily before meals. An extended-release formulation is also employed by some clinicians, usually as 75 mg taken once daily in the morning or midmorning. Both dosing regimens are effective in achieving short-term weight loss in excess of placebo. Complaints of insomnia increase if late afternoon dosing is used. Diethylpropion causes less CNS stimulation than Mazindol and generally causes less insomnia than phentermine. Patients with severe hypertension or significant cardiovascular disease should not receive diethylpropion. However, it is one of the safest noradrenergic appetite suppressants. This can be used in patients with mild to moderate hypertension or angina pectoris. Diabetic patients may experience decreased insulin or oral hypoglycemic dosage requirements soon after beginning therapy and prior to any substantial weight loss. More frequent blood glucose self-monitoring and medical follow-up is warranted when treating diabetic patients with diethylpropion.

Phenylpropanolamine

Although commonly classified as a noradrenergic anorexic, phenylpropanolamine (PPA) is atypical with regard to its mechanism and site of action. PPA racemers, D- and L-norephedrine, have chemical structures quite similar to amphetamine. PPA has been used for many years as a constituent of over-the-counter appetite suppressants and various cough and cold preparations. However, because of persistent case reports of hemorrhagic stroke related to PPA exposure, the United States Food and Drug Administration (FDA) and pharmaceutical manufacturers partnered to complete a case-control study known as The Hemorrhagic Stroke Project (HSP) during the 1990's. The final report of the HSP was submitted to the FDA in May 2000. In October 2000 The Nonprescription Drugs Advisory Committee discussed the HSP report and concluded that PPA is not safe for continued use. The FDA issued a public health warning in early November 2000 requesting that all manufacturers discontinue marketing of PPA-containing products.

Ephedrine

Chemically related to PPA (norephedrine), ephedrine may be a viable obesity pharmacotherapy agent. It appears to suppress appetite and increase energy expenditure via release of presynaptic norepinephrine and direct stimulation of thermogenic adrenergic receptors. The efficiency of ephedrine stimulation is somewhat blunted by physiologic feedback systems involving adenosine and various prostaglandins. This notion has stimulated research to characterize the effect of ephedrine in the presence of adenosine and prostaglandin antagonists such as caffeine and aspirin. Ephedrine in combination with caffeine has enhanced appetite suppression and thermogenesis as compared to placebo and other anorectics over time periods of up to 6 months. Oral doses of 20 mg ephedrine and 200 mg caffeine up to three times daily have been studied. The spectrum of side effects with ephedrine and ephedrine/caffeine combinations is similar to that seen with other noradrenergic agents. Side effects are more notable at higher doses and most commonly include tremor, agitation, nervousness, increased sweating, and insomnia; palpitations and tachycardia have also been reported. Patients with diabetes, hypertension, or cardiovascular disease (including arrhythmic conditions) should not self-medicate with ephedrine-containing products without evaluation by a qualified physician. Ephedrine is available both with and without a prescription; neither form is labeled by the FDA for use as an obesity therapy.

SEROTONERGIC AGENTS

Serotonin (5-HT) is an important neurotransmitter involved in many human physiologic systems. Sleep-wake cycle, sensitivity to pain, blood pressure, mood, and eating behaviors have links to serotonin activity. Increasing central serotonin levels decreases the amount of food consumed and prolongs the time between food intakes. Some serotonergic agents increase central serotonin concentrations via stimulating release of presynaptic stores and/or inhibition of reuptake into storage granules. Additionally, either the parent compound or metabolites of these agents may also directly stimulate postsynaptic 5-HT receptors. Peripheral serotonin effects that impact appetite, such as slowing gastric motility, have also been described. A major distinction between serotonergic and noradrenergic anorexiants is that serotonergic agents lack the central stimulant effects and abuse potential seen with the noradrenergic compounds. Conversely, decreased wakefulness, altered sleep patterns, and changes in affect can be seen.

ANTIDEPRESSANTS

Selective Serotonin Reuptake Inhibitors (SSRI). As a class, the serotonin reuptake inhibitors are generally weight-neutral as opposed to other commonly used compounds such as the tricyclic antidepressants. The National Task Force on the Prevention and Treatment of Obesity has reviewed multiple randomized, double-blinded, placebo-controlled weight-loss clinical trials using fluoxetine and sertraline. Patients receiving fluoxetine (60 mg/d) demonstrate initial weight loss of up to 2 to 4 kg on average, but weight regain occurs in spite of continued medication use such that no difference is noted between fluoxetine and placebo over periods of up to one year. Similar findings are noted using sertraline (200 mg/d) as an adjunct to help maintain weight lost with very low Calorie diet. A direct relationship exists between amount of weight lost and the sum of fluoxetine and (it's metabolite) norfluoxetine plasma concentrations. Higher plasma concentrations are associated with greater weight loss. The antidepressant serotonin reuptake inhibitors are not approved by the FDA as weight management agents and are not currently recommended for routine treatment of obesity. Some practitioners continue to prescribe these agents for the treatment of obesity, "off-label" either alone or in combination with phentermine. The safety and efficacy of phentermine-SSRI combinations are currently unclear. A case report of adverse experiences (impaired mentation, tremor, hyperreflexia, and gastrointestinal symptoms) with unintentional concurrent use of phentermine and fluoxetine reinforces the need for caution by prescribers of unlabeled combination therapy.

NORADRENERGIC/SEROTONERGIC AGENT

Sibutramine

An orally active racemic mixture, sibutramine became available in the United States in early 1998. The parent compound and two active metabolites (M_1 and M_2) appear to increase synaptic concentrations of serotonin (5-HT), norepinephrine (NE), and dopamine via reuptake inhibition. The active metabolites (M_1 and M_2) are more potent than the parent sibutramine. Reuptake inhibition appears to be greatest for norepinephrine, followed by serotonin, with dopamine the least inhibited.

Sibutramine has been studied in clinical trial in doses from 1-30 mg daily and demonstrates a relatively clear dose-response relationship. Weight loss from daily doses of 1 mg is, on average, no different than placebo. The recommended starting dose is 10 mg daily, with a recommended dose range of 5 to 15 mg daily. Dry mouth, anorexia, insomnia, constipation, appetite increase, dizziness, and nausea were noted two- to threefold more frequently in sibutramine-treated subjects than in placebo-treated subjects. Significant increases in both systolic and diastolic blood pressure and pulse rate have been noted with sibutramine use. Baseline blood pressure should be established prior to beginning therapy and close monitoring is required when using this agent. Sibutramine product labeling indicates that it should not be used in patients with a history of coronary artery disease, stroke, congestive heart failure, or arrhythmias. Like other centrally acting appetite suppressants, sibutramine should not be used by patients receiving MAO inhibitor therapies. Sibutramine is listed as a schedule IV prescription substance in spite of being noted as having no street value by recreational substance users. Primary pulmonary hypertension has not been reported with sibutramine use. Echocardiographic assessments of a small cohort of patients from clinical trials, with approximately 6 months exposure, do not demonstrate the cardiac valve problems seen with the fenfluramine derivatives. Based upon 12-month clinical trials, weight loss with sibutramine therapy appears to be most significant during the first 6 months of therapy. Twenty-nine percent of placebo-treated patients in these trials attained a 5% reduction in total body weight after 12 months. Using sibutramine at 10 and 15 mg/d resulted in 56% and 65% of patients, respectively, achieving at least a 5% reduction in total body weight. A 10% reduction in body weight was achieved by 8% of placebo-treated patients, while 30% and 39% of those taking sibutramine 10 and 15 mg/d, respectively, obtained this level of weight reduction. There is, on average, a tendency for weight regain after 6 months of treatment. As with other centrally active appetite suppressants, weight regain occurs with cessation of therapy. Safety and efficacy beyond one year of exposure to sibutramine are currently uncertain.

LIPASE INHIBITORS

Orlistat

The percentile of dietary intake as fat has been implicated as a contributing factor in the development of obesity. Fat represents an extremely dense energy source, providing 9 kcal/g as compared to approximately 4 kcal/g from protein or carbohydrate. In humans, most of accumulated body fat excess is derived from dietary sources because of a limited capacity to synthesize fat from carbohydrate. Gastrointestinal (gastric, pancreatic, and carboxylester) lipases are essential in the absorption of the long-chain triglycerides commonly found in Western diets. Additionally, lipase is known to play a role in facilitating gastric emptying and secretion of other pancreaticobiliary substances.

Orlistat (Xenical)

Orlistat is minimally absorbed and selectively inhibits gastrointestinal lipases. Lipases inhibition results in decreased formation of free fatty acids from dietary triglyceride. Additionally, lower luminal free fatty acid concentrations result in malabsorption of cholesterol. Orlistat induces weight loss by a persistent lowering of dietary fat absorption. Clinical studies employing orlistat as an adjunct to diet therapy demonstrated dose-dependent reductions in fat absorption.

No additional decrease in fat absorption occurs with doses above 400 mg/d. The drug must be taken with foods that contain fat in order to exert its effect. However, varying either meal content with regard to fat/fiber ratio or timing of drug ingestion relative to meal demonstrated little effect on the inhibition of fat absorption.

Soft stools, abdominal pain/colic, flatulence, fecal urgency, or incontinence is initially reported in up to 80% of individuals using orlistat. These complaints are most common in the first 1 to 2 months of therapy, are mild to moderate in severity, and tend to improve with continued use. Orlistat in addition to a low-calorie diet over a 1-year time period resulted in a small cohort of obese subjects who maintained a 7% to 9% decrease in body weight as opposed to placebo-treated subjects who experienced weight regain at 6 to 7 months of therapy. Orlistat-induced malabsorption of fat-soluble vitamins has been documented. Therefore, vitamin supplementation should be considered during therapy with this agent. Despite its definite effects on fat absorption and gastrointestinal motility, orlistat does not appear to change the pharmacokinetic or dynamic profiles of numerous other agents.

Results from a series of 1 to 2 year clinical trials indicate that this agent may prove to be an acceptable long-term medication supplement in medically supervised weight loss Programs. A 1-year, randomized, double-blind, placebo-controlled trial of orlistat in obese type 2 diabetics was completed. This trial demonstrated that prolonged use of orlistat results in significant sustainable weight loss with improvements in glycemic control and lipid profile. Orlistat use in addition to diet significantly promoted weight loss and less weight regain during another two-year, randomized, double-blind, placebo-controlled study. In this study, in addition to weight loss, orlistat use was associated with improvements in lipid profile and a sustained reduction in fasting insulin levels. Finally, a 2-year randomized, double-blind, placebo-controlled multicenter study completed in a primary care setting demonstrated similar outcomes with respect to orlistat utility as a supplement to medically supervised weight loss. Although unanimously recommended for approval by an FDA advisory committee in 1997, the FDA subsequently requested further information regarding the occurrence of breast cancer during clinical trials. An overall breast cancer incidence of 0.6% (nine cases, all female) was noted in the orlistat treatment versus 0.1% (one case, female) with placebo. In retrospect, evidence of malignancy prior to study participation was apparent in 8 of the 9 orlistat-treated patients. Clarification of this issue resulted in orlistat approval by the FDA in 1998, and its arrival in US markets in 1999.

Currently two drugs are used in the treatment of obesity:

1. Sibutanonine (Meridia), Dose: 5, 10, 15 mg. Start 10 mg po qd, may be increased to 15 mg or decreased to 5 mg.
   Adverse effects: tachycardia and increases in blood pressure
2. Oristat (Xenical), Dose: 120 mg po tid before meals
   Adverse effects: decrease in absorption of fat-soluble vitamins, soft stools and anal leakage

Only patients who are at increased medical risk because if they are overweight should use weight loss drugs.

N. HERBAL, NATURAL AND FOOD SUPPLEMENT WEIGHT LOSS THERAPIES

Many individuals choose to undertake weight loss regimens without medical monitoring that incorporate the ingestion of herbal, natural, or food supplement products. It is important to remember that the FDA does not strictly regulate the manufacture and labeling of these products.

Chromium

The inclusion of chromium as an effective agent for weight loss is unclear. The hexavalent form of this element is thought to be carcinogenic, while the trivalent form found in human food sources is essentially nontoxic. Chromium is considered an essential nutrient, and experimentally in animals is an insulin cofactor active in carbohydrate, protein, and lipid metabolism. In humans, insulin resistance has been reported in a few cases of apparent severe chromium deficiency during long-term total parenteral nutrition. Currently, there is no reliable means of assessing total body chromium status, making diagnosis of deficiency difficult. The tryptophan metabolite, picolinic acid, form a complex with trivalent chromium, which improves bioavailability. Food sources with highly available chromium include brewer's yeast, calf liver, American cheese, and wheat germ. A double-blind, placebo-controlled study of chromium picolinate as a supplement to aerobic exercise in the treatment of obesity failed to demonstrate any effectiveness.

St. John's Wort

A perennial flowering plant (Hypericum perforatum), St. John's Wort has been employed as a medicinal herb for thousands of years. Its use in weight loss and herbal supplements is probably based upon the proposed effects of its constituent naphthodianthrones (hypericin and pseudohypericin). These are thought to be inhibitors of monoamine oxidase, and would be expected to increase synaptic concentrations of monoamines such as serotonin and norepinephrine. Consistent with these assumptions, hypericum extracts appear to be more effective than placebo in the treatment of depression. However, *in vitro* studies have not been able to substantiate direct monoamine oxidase inhibition at physiologic hypericin concentrations and recognized antidepressant effects may be due to other constituents. The risks of concurrent use of Hypericum derivatives and other adrenergic and serotonergic compounds have not been characterized. Currently, St. John's Wort has not been studied with respect to its role in obesity management, and its safety and efficacy as a treatment modality in the self-management of obesity are unclear.

Chitosan
Chitosan is a cationic polysaccharide, specifically, a partially N-deacetylated form of chitin. This nonhydrolyzable fiber exhibits properties similar to cellulose. *In vitro* and pre-clinical data has indicated that chitosan may be effective in blocking absorption of fat from the gut. It has been suggested that orally administered chitosan may be an effective weight reduction agent by blocking calories ingested as fat. Chitosan is a major constituent in several heavily advertised weight management food supplements and over-the-counter preparation. However, a small number of properly randomized and blinded or open-label investigations currently demonstrate that orally administered chitosan is not an effective inhibitor of fat absorption in humans. Additionally, head-to-head comparisons of chitosan versus orlistat have been completed. These investigations clearly demonstrate that orlistat blocks 30-50% of ingested fat versus negligible effects with chitosan. While further research may be warranted with respect to the appropriate dose in humans needed to impair fat absorption, current claims of chitosan effectiveness in humans are unsubstantiated.

O. COMMERCIAL WEIGHT LOSS PROGRAMS

These programs are generally conducted without medical supervision and may not provide dietary guidance. These programs may include meal replacements, vitamins, and dietary supplements. Some of these programs can be safe if dietary guidelines are followed. Data on the efficacy of these commercial weight loss programs indicate successful short-term weight loss for some participants. Some adverse effects like, arrhythmias, gallstones, have been associated with some herbal remedies.

COMBINATION THERAPY

Diet Therapy + Exercise + Behavior Modification
This therapy is the best in the treatment of overweight and obesity. Several studies have shown that combination of low Calorie diet, regular physical activity and behavior modification suited for individual's life style produce best results.

Diet Therapy + Exercise + Behavior Modification + Meal Replacement
Sometimes the physician may recommend one meal replacement. The replacement may be for breakfast, lunch, dinner or in between snack. This may be recommended if the patient's life style does not permit to

take three meals and the patient is moving constantly. It may be also recommended if the patient is having problems with portion sizes.

Diet Therapy + Exercise + Behavior Modification + Drug Therapy
This combination therapy can be useful for patients with BMI of ≥ 30, and those who have failed with traditional weight loss program. Drug therapy combined with behavioral counseling, diet therapy, and exercise can be beneficial for some obese patients. The common drugs used include Sibutramine and Orlistat.

P. INDIVIDUALIZED WEIGHT REDUCTION PROGRAM

Weight reduction program should be tailor made to the needs of the patient. Large individual variation exists with any social or cultural group. Obesity treatment programs must be culturally sensitive. Some of the things that a physician should take into account when designing a weight reduction program for the patient include:

1. **Rate of Weight Loss. Following things should be assessed:**
   - present weight of the patient
   - medical problems
   - prescribed and over the counter medications patients may be taking that might cause weight gain
   - life style – this may influence how the patient incorporates diet therapy and physical activity
   - family support
   - motivation – the rate at which the patient feels comfortable to lose weight. Some patients may not be able to do much physical activity because of some medical problems like, asthma, arthritis, etc. In this case the weight loss will be slower.

2. **Identify common eating problems:**
   - meal skipping
   - sweet foods
   - salty foods
   - lack of flexibility
   - alcohol consumption
   - eating out frequently
   - night eaters
   - cleaning the plate
   - snacking all the time

Q. RECOMMENDATIONS FOR INDIVIDUALIZING WEIGHT REDUCTION PROGRAM

1. Set the goal and rate of losing weight with the patient.
2. Identify the type of eater and accordingly initiate behavior modification guidelines as discussed earlier.
3. Plan the diet in consultation with the patient taking into account his/her likes, dislikes, allergies, availability of foods, family dynamics and the medication the patient is currently taking.
4. Physical Activity. Discuss with the patient whether he/she is doing any exercise at the present time and whether they have any medical problems that will prevent the patient from doing intensive program. Physicians may get them started on low level activity.
5. Follow-up Visit. This is very important. Frequency may be decided in consultation with the patient. Overweight/obesity is a chronic condition and it should be monitored regularly.

R. MAINTENANCE

Communication between patient and physician is very important in maintaining motivation and commitment to weight maintenance. Counseling for successful maintenance of weight loss should focus on the following factors:

1. Regular visits to the physician's office. The visits can be short and they may be every two weeks or once a month. If the physician is busy, nurse can weigh in the patient.
2. Pairing up patients so that they can talk and help each other can also be useful.
3. Dietary composition. The maintenance stage can be more difficult for patients because the energy requirements are even lower than during the weight loss period. There is a reduced resting metabolic rate and a reduced rate of fat oxidation. To adjust to these metabolic changes, the diet needs to be very low in total calories and low in fat.
4. Physical Activity. Physical activity is particularly beneficial to the maintenance of weight loss. Research has shown combination of diet and exercise is very important in maintaining the weight.
5. Booster Sessions during a 3-month post-treatment period.
6. Inclusion of a significant other in the treatment.

S. SURGERY

Morbid obesity is a problem with its greatest prevalence in the United States (seven million people; 2% of men, 6% of women). It is defined as being 100 lbs over "**ideal body weight**" or weight approaching these levels but is complicated by multiple obesity-related health issues such as degenerative joint disease, diabetes (present in 34%), hyperlipidemia (40%), hypertension (46%), gout, gallstones, thromboembolism, lower extremity edema, obstructive sleep apnea (22% or more), and hepatic steatosis. Severe obesity is associated with a mortality rate at least double, and possibly, 6 to 12 times that of the nonobese [17, 18].

Medical treatment for severe obesity with various diets, psychotherapy, behavioral modification, pharmacotherapy and exercise, either alone or in combination, has been disappointing with little successful long-term weight reduction. Low Calorie diet programs can often result in rather dramatic short-term weight reduction but offers dismal long-term results. Pharmacotherapy typically only results in at best a 15% weight reduction which is inadequate for severely obese patients. Thus, the National Institutes of Health Consensus conference on obesity surgery suggested that patients with a BMI >40 kg/M^2 or those with BMI >35 kg/M^2 and with serious medical problems should be considered candidates for surgical intervention. Typically patients, who are by this definition morbidly overweight, should also have shown "reasonable attempts" to loose weight and have had a thorough psychological evaluation before being considered candidates for bariatric surgery. All patients need to understand the responsibilities of bariatric surgery before the surgery especially regarding life-long changes in diet, exercise, lifestyle and the long-term need for behavioral intervention.

Gastric Restrictive Procedure – Vertical Banded Gastroplasty

Vertical Banded Gastroplasty (VBG) is a purely restrictive procedure. In this procedure the upper stomach near the esophagus is stapled vertically for about 2-1/2 inches (6 cm) to create a smaller stomach pouch. The outlet from the pouch is restricted by a band or ring that slows the emptying of the food and thus creates the feeling of fullness.

Advantages:

- The primary advantage of this restrictive procedure is that a reduced amount of well-chewed food enters and passes through the digestive tract in the usual order. That allows the nutrients and vitamins (as well as the calories) to be fully absorbed into the body.

- After 10 years, studies show that patients can maintain 50% of targeted excess weight loss.

Risks:

- Postoperatively, stapling of the stomach carries with it the risk of staple-line disruption that can result in leakage and/or serious infection. This may require prolonged hospitalization with antibiotic treatment and/or additional operations.
- Staple-line disruption may also, in the long-term, lead to weight gain. For these reasons, some surgeons divide the staple-line wall of the pouch from the rest of the stomach to reduce the risk of long-term staple-line disruption.
- The band or ring applied may lead to complications of obstruction or perforation, requiring surgical intervention.
- Characteristically, these procedures, while creating a sense of fullness, do not provide the necessary feeling of satisfaction that one has had "enough" to eat.
- Because restrictive procedures relay solely on a small pouch to reduce food intake, there is the risk of the pouch stretching or of the restricting band or ring at the pouch outlet breaking or migrating, thus allowing patients to eat too much.
- Around 40% of patients undergoing these procedures have lost less than half their excess body weight.
- As is the case with all weight loss surgeries, readmission to a hospital may be require for fluid replacement or nutritional support if there is excessive vomiting and adequate food intake cannot be maintained.

While these operations also reduce the size of the stomach, the stomach pouch created is much larger than with other procedures. The goal is to restrict the amount of food consumed and alter the normal digestive process, but to a much greater degree. The anatomy of the small intestine is changed to divert the bile and pancreatic juices so they meet the ingested food closer to the middle or the end of the small intestine. With the three approaches discussed below, absorption of nutrients and calories is also reduced, but to a much greater degree than with previously discussed procedures. Each of the three differs in how and when the digestive juices (i.e., bile) come into contact with the food.

Since food bypasses the duodenum, all the risk considerations discussed in the gastric bypass section regarding the malabsorption of some minerals and vitamins also apply to these techniques, only to greater degree.

Other Surgical Procedures:

Biliopancreatic Diversion (BPD). BPD removes approximately ¾ of the stomach to produce both restriction of food intake and reduction of acid output. Leaving enough upper stomach is important to maintain proper nutrition. The small intestine is then divided with one end attached to the stomach pouch to create what is called an "alimentary limb." All the food moves through this segment, however, not much is absorbed. The bile and pancreatic juices move through the biliopancreatic limb," which is connected to the side of the intestine close to the end. This supplies digestive juice in the section of the intestine now called the "common limb." The surgeon is able to vary the length of the common limb to regulate the amount of absorption of protein, fat, and fat-soluble vitamins.

Extended (Distal) Roux-en-Y Gastric Bypass (RYGBP-E). RYGBP-E is an alternative means of achieving malabsorption by creating a stapled or divided small gastric pouch, leaving the remainder of stomach in place. A long limb of the small intestine is attached to the stomach to divert the bile and pancreatic juices. This procedure carries with it fewer operative risks by avoiding removal of the lower ¾ of the stomach. Gastric pouch size and the length of the bypassed intestine determine the risks for ulcers, malnutrition, and other effects.

Biliopancreatic Diversion with "Duodenal Switch". This procedure is a variation of BPD in which stomach removal is restricted to the outer margin, leaving a sleeve of stomach with the pylorus and the beginning of the duodenum at its end. The duodenum, the first portion of the small intestine, is divided so that pancreatic and bile drainage is bypassed. The near end of the "alimentary limb" is then attached to the beginning of the duodenum, while the "common limb" is created in the same way as described above.

Bariatric surgery is primarily designed to help reduce food intake and thus caloric consumption. Various types of surgeries have been developed over the years which have reduced the size of the stomach (gastroplasty) in several different fashions which can be used in conjunction with increasing degrees of small intestinal bypass. The first surgery for obesity was developed in the early 1950's and did not involve the stomach. The jejunoileal bypass essentially induced malabsorption by connecting 35 cm of proximal jejunum to the distal 10 cm of the ileum. Since little absorptive area is left for food, it obviously requires very little patient compliance, but is associated with many complications including death (4%), hepatic cirrhosis and liver failure, immune complex arthritis (18%), kidney stones (nephrocalcinosis; 7% oxalate stones), chronic severe diarrhea (62%), and many electrolyte (hypokalemia, hypocalcemia, hypomagnesemia) imbalances (58%), vitamin (vitamin D in 43%) and mineral deficiencies. It appears many of these complications were due to the bacterial overgrowth which developed in the blind loop.

Why weight loss occurs in gastric bypass is unknown. It had originally been thought to be due to a slowing of gastric emptying (satiety increased) and the dumping syndrome (nausea, weakness, sweating, palpitations, faintness, postprandial diarrhea). But neither correlates to the weight loss. As a matter of fact, liquids typically have a faster emptying after bypass surgery. In addition, gastric bypass has been shown to be more effective than gastroplasty.

Since the risk of developing gallstones is very high after a weight reduction surgery (36%), a prophylactic cholecystectomy is routinely performed with bariatric surgery. About 30% of patients undergoing such surgery will already have gallstones present at the time of the surgery.

Recently, laparoscopic gastric banding has been suggested as a less invasive means to cause gastric reduction. The technique places a band around the upper portion of the stomach. Even laparoscopic gastric bypass surgery is now being performed but requires more than double the surgical time (four hours) than conventional bypass surgery. Long-term studies are still needed to assess the clinical usefulness of these procedures.

It is important that each patient who is being considered for bariatric surgery is evaluated not only by the surgeon but a nutritionist, dietitian and behavioral psychologist. A good preoperative assessment can reduce significantly postoperative complications and problems. It is very important that every patient undergo a thorough history and physical which assess for the medical complications of obesity with particular attention to the presence of obstructive sleep apnea. Sleep apnea is a serious and life-threatening condition which can cause cardiac arrhythmias and heart failure. An electrocardiogram should be done, obviously looking for signs of cardiac disease, but also eliminating the presence of a prolong QT interval which has been associated with an increased risk of sudden death in the postoperative period and during rapid weight loss.

Psychological testing and evaluation should screen for substance abuse, significant eating disorder (e.g. bulimia), major psychiatric illness, and psychosocial stressors which may impair successful compliance with post-operative care. Active substance abuse, schizophrenia, borderline personality disorder, and uncontrolled depression should be considered an absolute contraindication for surgery. Some studies have found the prevalence of binge eating disorder, bulimia nervosa, night eating syndrome and drinking large quantities of fluids very common in bariatric surgery patients and such behaviors typically remain unaltered after surgery.

Although age should not be considered a contraindication to bariatric surgery, often other concurrent medical problems need to be assessed such as diabetes, cardiopulmonary disease and previous abdominal surgeries which might adversely affect the postoperative course. In addition, all patients must fully understand the surgical procedure and implications for permanently changing one's eating and activity habits. This is not simply a procedure to anatomically change the gastrointestinal tract but a procedure which should permanently alter one's lifestyle to one conducive of a healthy body weight and a lifestyle of healthy eating and exercise. Success is typically defined as loosing 50% or more of the excess body weight and not reaching "ideal body weight". Realistic expectations must be comprehended by all surgical candidates. Sometimes success is in other terms such as the resolution of health issues and improved quality of life. This is a major commitment not just to the surgery, but to taking nutritional supplements adhering to proper dietary guidelines, regular exercise and returning for scheduled post-operative visits. Only through a team or multidisciplinary approach will the post-surgical course of the patient be optimized towards a successful outcome.

All candidates for surgery should understand and acknowledge the severity of their obesity and its associated complications. A presurgical inventory of dietary compliance may help in assessing postoperative compliance or at least assess needed areas of education or behavioral intervention. Other signs of good compliance are the ability to stop smoking and keep medical appointments.

Severe obesity increases the risk for post-operative pneumonia or atelectasis. Incentive spirometry has been shown to decrease such complications after abdominal surgery. Risk for deep venous thrombosis is also increased in morbidly obese patients. Yet, the most effective way to reduce this is using Thrombo-Gards when in bed and ambulating the patient as soon as possible after the surgery. Death is an uncommon event after gastric surgery (<1%). Incisional infections occur in 5% of individuals. Dehiscence wound is even more uncommon, less likely is an anastomotic leak. When leaks occur, typically they will heal on their own with time, only rarely requiring reoperation. Nausea and vomiting occurs in 10% of patients but typically subsides in most patients by three months. When this continues, worsens, or reoccurs, then an evaluation for stomach complications should be done using endoscopy. If this is negative, assessment for a formal eating disorder should be conducted.

It is typical for most patients to loose 0.5 to 1 pound daily for the first three months, half this rarely the second three months and 3-5 pounds over a week or less the remainder of the first year after surgery. Most patients typically stabilize by 12 to 18 months after the surgery, losing 50-60% of their excess body weight. Continued weight reduction requires continued efforts at lifestyle modification, diet modification, and an active exercise program. Weight loss should not be the main focus of a patient's success. The resolution of the patient's weight-related comorbidities is more important.

During this period of active weight loss, it is not uncommon for patients to complain of fatigue (flu-like symptoms), feeling cold when others feel comfortable, dry skin and hair thinning. These typically resolve with time as the weight loss slows and eventually plateaus. Over 70% of patients will loose more than 50% of their excess body weight and keep this off for five years after the bariatric bypass surgery.

Diet after Gastric Surgery

In general, the diet following gastric surgery limits beverages and liquids at meals and the intake of simple carbohydrates, is high in protein and moderate in fat, and avoids foods that are known to increase intestinal peristalsis, such as caffeine. Small, frequent feedings should be provided initially. If no complications occur, additional foods are added as tolerated. Some patients are able to advance to a general diet within 2 to 3 weeks. After gastric surgery, the diet generally progresses as follows:

- Ice chips are allowed 24 to 48 hours after surgery or small, infrequent sips of water are given. Some people tolerate warm water better than ice chips or cold water.
- Clear liquids such as broth, bouillon, unsweetened gelatin, or diluted unsweetened fruit juices are given.
- The postgastrectomy diet can be initiated with gradual progression to a general diet as tolerated. Solid foods (limiting caffeine, acidic foods, peppermint, and chocolate) can be started, but a more important priority is offering the patient foods that are liked and well tolerated. By the 4th or 5th day, many patients can tolerate solid foods. Some patient may experience dumping syndrome following surgery.
- High-fat foods are limited. Patients with partial gastric resection frequently have mild fat malabsorption.

The adequacy of the diet depends on the extent of surgery as well as individual food tolerance. With careful selection, this diet is adequate in all nutrients.

The diarrhea, which is usually postprandial, can typically be treated with loperamide or diphenoxylate which reduces the incidence of the diarrhea by about 50%. It is not uncommon that certain foods are difficult to tolerate (high sugar, fat and fiber) even months and years after the surgery. The "dumping syndrome" initially acts as an aid in restricting eating after surgery and usually disappears within 12 to 18 months. Yet, continued periodic challenges of healthy food items are encouraged since often these "intolerances" resolve with bowel adaptation. On rare occasions, reactive hypoglycemia can occur. This is more common when a diet high in simple sugars is consumed and classic hypoglycemic symptoms occur within 4-5 hours of the meal and a measured plasma glucose level is less than 55 mg/dl during the symptoms. Usually better dietary habits will resolve this but on occasion treatment with Acarbose, 25 mg with each meal, will delay carbohydrate absorption enough to control such episodes of hypoglycemia.

The symptoms of dumping syndrome can be complicated by symptoms of lactose intolerance, depending on the extent of intestinal mucosa resected. A secondary lactace deficiency can result in symptoms similar to those seen in dumping syndrome. Therefore, milk products should be introduced slowly to determine tolerance. Dried fat-free milk or various caseins are generally well tolerated. A lactose tolerance test or breath hydrogen test can be performed to diagnose a lactase deficiency. Malabsorption of calcium and vitamin D may lead to the development of osteomalacia. Persons with minimal or no intake of milk or dairy products may need vitamin D and calcium supplementation. If milk intolerance is caused by lactose intolerance, various lactose-free commercial formulas with high-calorie, high-protein densities and low osmolatities are available. Lactose-reduced milk may be tolerated because lactase enzymes simply reduce disaccharides to mono-saccharides, which are just as likely to promote dumping syndrome.

In persons who have had a partial or total gastrectomy or vagotomy, hypoglycemia may occur 1 to 2 hours following meals. The rapid digestion and absorption of foods causes an elevation of blood glucose, which leads to over-production of insulin and subsequent hypoglycemia. Symptoms of hypoglycemia include weakness, nausea, perspiration, hunger, anxiety, and tremors. To prevent hypoglycemia, patients should avoid simple carbohydrates such as candy, sugar, jam, jelly, syrup, honey, cola drinks, cookies, cakes, and ice cream unless made with sugar substitutes. Simple forms of sugar should be consumed only for treatment of hypoglycemia. A protein source should be included with each meal.

Many patients will incur in time the same weight regain. Most commonly, old unhealthy lifestyle habits return, whether this be reduction in activity or falling back to old eating habits. Control lies in returning back to basic principles of using food records and exercise (activity) log books. This is often a time when a behavioral psychologist can be helpful in trying to assist the patient to identify stressors or recent life obstacles which have contributed to the weight regain.

However, if appetite control is the issue, this is one of the few occasions where pharmacotherapy may indeed be useful. These patients have been through a major surgical procedure and maintaining their weight loss should be treated aggressively. Obviously, each patient requires a thorough evaluation of the causes of the weight regain before using appetite suppressants. Appetite suppressant, sibutramine (Meridia) at 10 mg daily and can be increased to a maximal dose of 15 mg a day as tolerated. Unlike fenfluramine and dexfenfluramine, which increased serotonin levels in the brain by increasing serotonin secretion, this drug affects serotonin and norepinephrine reuptake. No valvular damage has been reported with this drug at present. However, the drug can cause significant increase in blood pressure and all patients should be monitored closely for such changes. Other side effects include dry mouth, insomnia and constipation. Typically it causes a 5-10% weight loss, but studies have not been done using this drug in post-bariatric surgery patients. At present, it would be the drug of choice for controlling appetite if this problem arises. If the problem is more consistent with an eating disorder like bulimia, then fluoxetine (Prozac) and sertraline (Zoloft) have been shown to be helpful in controlling binge eating.

Health improvements often occur very quickly after gastric bypass surgery. Lipid levels decrease 20-50%, 90% of Type II diabetes resolves, hypertension resolves in 66%, and sleep apnea is cured in 40% of patients who have had these problems preoperatively. Gastroesophageal reflux is typically resolved with the Roux-en-Y procedure but is often worsen or unaffected by gastroplasty. Other health benefits include improved urinary incontinence in women, less pain from degenerative joint disease (or capable of undergoing joint replacement in severely advanced DJD) and psychological functioning. This improvement in health plus the changes in body size leads to an overall improved quality of life. Sometimes the most remarkable changes occur in the ability of the patients to pursue normal activities of daily life.

However, several complications may occur. It is the physician's responsibility to screen for these and to prevent them when possible. Stomach ulcers occur in 5% of patients and typically present as abdominal pain or gastrointestinal bleeding. Typically this can be controlled with omeprazole or other "anti-ulcer" medications. Rarely a stricture can develop at the ancestomotie site which typically responds to endoscopic dilatation. Surgery is rarely necessary for either complication.

Abdominal and incisional hernias are very common (10%). This typically requires repair but is reserved to when the patient has reached nadir weight or if symptoms necessitate an earlier repair. Obviously, redundant abdominal wall tissue can present as a site of chronic superficial ulceration and infection necessitating a removal of the pannus. Other sites requiring such skin fold reductions include the upper arms, neck, buttocks, and thighs.

More commonly vitamin B12 deficiency will occur in those patients not routinely instructed in the administration of parenteral B12 administration after Roux-en-Y gastric bypass surgery. It is more cost effective to begin vitamin B12 administration after surgery than to rely on repetitive measurements of B12 levels.

More than 50% of patients will require iron supplementation. This is more common in menstruating woman than other patients and is usually assessed by iron studies (iron, TIBC) at 6 months and one year postoperatively. The iron deficiency develops for two reasons; one is the obvious continued loss of iron in menstruating females but the lack of absorption of iron due to bypassing the duodenum the major site for iron absorption, as well as the loss of the acid melieu necessary for iron absorption (conversion of dietary iron from the ferrous to ferric state).

Calcium metabolism is similarly disturbed in patients after a Roux-en-Y procedure. Once again the duodenum is the major site for calcium absorption. Recent studies have suggested that bariatric surgery may be a major risk factor for the development of osteoporosis. In some patients, especially patients with long limb bypasses, osteomalacia develops from Vitamin D deficiency. Obese individuals have lower vitamin D levels preoperatively, and these can become lower after by-pass surgery causing elevation in parathyroid hormone which can lead to osteomalacia. During follow up assessments, any elevation in alkaline phosphatase enzymes should be appropriately investigated for possibly vitamin D deficiency. If vitamin D deficiency occurs, treatment is typically oral administration of 25-OH vitamin D at 50,000 units one to two times a week. Only rarely does this necessitate parenteral supplementation.

Bariatric surgery patients are at a much higher risk for osteoporosis. This is without findings of vitamin D deficiency, hypocalcemia, hypocalciuria, or secondary hyperparathyroidism. The etiology of this remains undetermined but may be related to both the rate of weight loss and the marked degree of impaired intestinal calcium absorption. Further studies are needed in this area.

In very long limb bypass surgeries and more commonly, in partial pancreaticobiliary bypass, other malabsorptive syndromes can occur. Deficiencies in magnesium, zinc, selenium, vitamins A, E (rarely K) can occur and require long-term supplementation. Most patients have persistent and frequent diarrhea, however, this is not always the case.

The fat soluble vitamins can present in different manners. Vitamin D deficiency as discussed above, usually presents with signs and symptoms of osteomalacia but can also cause psychiatric manifestations, renal tubular proteinuria and neuropathy. Vitamin A deficiency most commonly presents with loss of night vision, but other visual complaints can predominate (xerophthalmia) as well as skin and mucous membrane changes. Vitamin E deficiency can cause anemia, ophthalmoplegia, and peripheral neuropathy. Vitamin K deficiency is rare, but typically presents with easy bruising, and bleeding tendencies.

If deficiencies in these vitamins develop, replacement therapies start at 5,000 to 10,000 IU of vitamin A orally daily; 50,000 IU of vitamin D2 (ergosterol) orally 1-3 times per week (or 1 cc of ergosterol in sesame oil (500,000 IU/ml) per month); 800 RU of vitamin E orally daily and 10 mg of vitamin K injected SQ daily until prothrombin time is normalized then 10 mg orally (daily) thereafter. Follow up of these levels is necessary to determine the correct replacement dosage acutely and chronically. Levels can change as the bowel adaptation occurs as well.

Trace element deficiencies typically do not present with signs and symptoms but are usually discovered by checking their levels after the above vitamin levels are found deficient or chronic severe diarrhea persists more than a few months. Zinc deficiency can cause rashes, alopecia, and lethargy. Magnesium deficiency can cause palpitations, arrthythmias, hypocalceniia, muscular twitching, numbness, tingling and a positive Chvostek and Trousseau's signs. Selenium deficiency rarely presents with cardiomyopathy. When trace element deficiencies are found, magnesium is corrected by using magnesium oxide 600 mg tablets (360 mg of elemental Mg) orally 1-3 times daily. Magnesium can decrease the absorption of digoxin, tetracycline and quinolones. Also, calcium supplementation to more than 2.6 grams per day can lead to negative magnesium balance, thus both urinary calcium and magnesium levels may need to be followed for adequate replacement. There are also several other types of magnesium which can be used for replacement if the oxide is not tolerated (e.g. gluconate). Zinc replacement is typically with 67 mg zinc sulfate tablets given orally 1-3 times daily. High doses of zinc can cause copper deficiency especially when given long-term. Selenium can be replaced by 100 to 200 micrograms orally.

Medication absorption can also be disturbed most particularly after long limb bypasses. Oral contraceptives may not be reliable under these conditions. It is not uncommon to see patients requiring much higher and divided doses of thyroid replacement hormone. Other medications may be likewise affected (e.g. Digoxin, Dilantin).

Intestinal adaptation is greater in the ileum than jejunum with increased length and thickness occurring with hyperplasia and increased villous height. This adaptation appears to affect gastrointestinal symptoms, food intolerances and even weight loss. This may be a major contributor to the 22-50% weight regain in the five years following the minimum weight achieved after such surgery.

Typically the patients are seen every three months during the first year after surgery and annually thereafter by a physician/nutritionist. Visits with the dietitian and behavioral psychologist are more frequent in the first year and long-term behavioral intervention is recommended for most patients. All patients are required to take a multivitamin (two chewable children vitamins until one to two adult tablets such as Theragram-M or equivalent is tolerated), 1,500-2,000 mg of calcium daily, and monthly vitamin B12 injections (educated in self-injection). Maintaining compliance with these supplements, dietary guidelines and a daily exercise program is a critical part of each patient's postsurgical care.

During the physician encounters, it is common to have a complete blood count (CBC), serum sodium, potassium, calcium, phosphorus, creatinine, glucose (glycosylated hemoglobin level if diabetes was present preoperatively), liver function tests (AST, alkaline phosphatase, bilirubin) and albumin levels measured. At six and twelve months postoperatively, iron and TIBC levels are measured. Special tests for vitamin and trace elements are only done if indicated by patients' symptoms or blood test results. For example, an elevated alkaline phosphatase level would lead to the measurement of isoenzymes. If the bone fraction is elevated, then 25-OH-vitamin D levels are measured. If one fat soluble vitamin is found deficient then the others are typically checked as well as serum magnesium, zinc and selenium levels. Clinical judgment is important in choosing the right tests and a thorough medical history at each visit will assist in the clinicians' medical assessment of the patient regarding the possibility of such deficiencies.

Many psychological issues can arise after surgery. Anxiety and depression over a longer than expected "recovery period" is common. The development of an "eating disorder" or the uncovering of previously unrecognized eating disorders can appear. Typically patients have unrealistic expectations about the effect of surgery on relationships, sex and work. The patient may lose friends, have sexual problems and be treated differently at work and socially. This emphasizes the importance of professional counseling before and after bariatric surgery.

Often, significant weight loss leads to changes in interpersonal relationships. Marital discord can occur as the body image of the patient changes dramatically along with the social responses to the patient. This can not only be stressful to the patient but also to the patient's spouse or family. At times, this often "liberates" the patient from past inhibitions and such changes can result in new social stressors.

Most studies seem to show patients to be more physically and socially active 6 months after surgery. Unemployment decreases 20-40%. Better sexual satisfaction has been described. However, increased tobacco and alcohol abuse has been observed as well as an increased dissatisfaction with the patient's spouse. Divorce rates are higher three years after surgery but are obviously more common in marriages with dysfunction preoperatively.

Much psychological support is necessary either individually or in group programs. All patients should be minimally involved in a supportive group programs, if not, individual meetings with a psychologist with experience in this area, in hopes to identify these issues and others which may interfere with the long-term successful outcome of the surgery on the patient's health.

Often redundant skin and a marked abdominal panniculus is a result of the massive weight loss secondary to bariatric surgery. Plastic surgery is only advised once the weight has stabilized for 1-2 years. This is often considered a cosmetic surgery by third party payers unless as abdominal panniculus is complicated by infection or ulceration. If this occurs, it should be clearly documented to allow patients financial assistance for this needed surgery. Often these surgeries are done in conjunction with abdominal hernia repair.

Occasionally, suction-assisted lipectomy or liposuction, what is now called liposculpture, is occasionally done in the post-bypass patient who desires further contouring. Surgical lipectomy is often applied to sites such as the upper arms, breasts, thighs and axillae.

T. RELAPSE PREVENTION

In weight control, a relapse can occur either during the weight-loss process, when someone who has made a commitment to a weight-loss program fails to adhere to its dietary prescriptions and fails to lose weight or after weight loss has occurred. In the latter situation, relapse can be considered a weight regain.

The term relapse might best be understood in relation to its opposite: maintenance of weight loss. Maintenance can be defined as weight loss that is kept off over time. Conversely, a relapse can be defined as weight loss that is subsequently regained.

These definitions are difficult to quantify. How long must weight loss be kept off to be considered maintained? How much weight must be regained to be considered a relapse? No general agreement exists as to how to quantify these constructs, and the literature contains numerous definitions utilized by different investigators. These definitions include:

- **Successful losers**: individuals who lost 20 or more pounds and kept it off for a year or longer.
- **Regainers**: individuals who lost weight, but regained 20% or more.
- **Maintainers**: individuals who regained less than 20%.
- **Poor maintainers**: individuals who regained more than 50% of weight previously lost.
- **Good maintainers**: individuals who regain less than 30% of weight previously lost.

These definitions, chosen by the investigators, may not correspond with the dieter's own perception of success or failure at maintenance. Few if any reported studies have asked dieters to assess their own levels of success. Yet it is likely that individuals differ in their subjective assessments of success and failure. Two individuals who have each lost 30 pounds and regained 10 pounds, for example, may differ in satisfaction with their performance. This difference may affect feelings of self-efficacy, which can in turn affect future performance. Perception of oneself as successful (especially if success is perceived as resulting from one's own skills rather than from chance or some external source) may lead to enhanced self-efficacy and continued effort directed toward weight loss or maintenance.

A final definition of relapse is based upon the common assumption that changes in target behaviors such as rate and amount of food consumed lead to weight loss. These target behaviors function as rules governing eating. Accepting this assumption, maintenance could be defined as continued use of rules governing eating behavior. Relapse could be considered the violation of one or more such rules. Asking dieters to state the techniques they have used most frequently during weight loss, and examining levels of continued adherence to these techniques after weight loss, could potentially provide valuable information about the role of target behaviors in the maintenance-relapse process. Behaviors critical for maintenance may differ from those critical for weight loss.

A dieter will follow a set of rules that govern eating and exercise behavior until he/she encounters high-risk situation. High-risk situations found to be especially prevalent among dieters include negative states such as boredom and depression and positive states occurring in social situations such as parties. If the dieter does not cope effectively and eat more food than is consistent with his/her weight-loss or maintenance goals, they may not have the skills needed to cope adequately in the high-risk situation. Numerous factors are involved in the maintenance process. Adherence to changes in diet and exercise patterns can be accomplished by self-monitoring and other behavior modification changes. Another important factor in making positive changes is the inclusion of significant others in treatment.

The relapse rate in weight reduction programs is very high. Approximately two-thirds of all relapses occur within the first 90 days following treatment. The relapse prevention program should include discussion of:

1. Analysis of high-risk situations
2. Ways of handling slips
3. Abstinence violation effect
4. Focus on long-term maintenance of weight loss
5. Coping strategies used by dieters in high-risk situations

Matching the Diet to the Lifestyle of the Patient

Weight management for treating obesity includes dietary modifications, physical activity, and behavioral intervention. Treatment should be adapted to the circumstances of each patient. No single approach is appropriate for all obese patients. The emphasis that is placed on diet, exercise, and behavioral interventions varies among individuals.

When counseling an obese patient for weight reduction, it is important to individual's dietary recommendations, based on the patient's current eating habits, lifestyle, ethnicity and culture, other coexisting medical conditions, and potential nutrition-medication interactions. In general, diet recommendations for weight loss include calorie reduction with attention to limiting portion sizes, avoid skipping meals with a minimum of three meals per day, reducing fat intake and emphasizing on more complex carbohydrates. It is recommended to include a variety of foods daily since no one food provides all the nutrients the body needs. Therefore, encourage patient to eat a variety of vegetables, fruits, whole grains, meat, and low fat diary products to optimize nutrition. Also, foods with higher fiber and/or water content such as fresh fruits, vegetables, and whole grains can help weight loss efforts by providing a sense of satiety-fullness-due to adding volume without the addition of extra calories.

For most patients, a moderate caloric restriction that is equal or near to the estimated basal energy expenditure is sufficient for weight loss. By creating an energy deficit of 500-1000 kcal/day, a rate of weight loss of 1 to 2 pounds per week could be achieved, depending on the activity level of the patient. A moderate weight loss over a longer period of time is recommended rather than to regain weight from a marked weight loss which is counterproductive. The calorie level can be adjusted depending on weight changes, intolerance to the current calorie level (i.e., feeling too hungry), and to halt any further weight loss if weight maintenance is indicated.

To assist a patient in changing dietary and activity habits, counseling needs to focus on a lifestyle approach. Setting realistic goals of current behaviors to modify related to eating and exercise is beneficial for weight management. Goals related to eating behaviors might include not skipping meals, consuming smaller meals, eating slowly, or separating food consumption from other activities. Self-monitoring of eating and exercise behaviors is also recommended. Recording dietary intake (food choices, amounts, meal times and caloric intake) and physical activity (mode of exercise, time, duration) can help with changing the behavior in the desired direction. Self-monitoring of weight is also important for long-term maintenance.

Research suggests that long-term treatment for weight management is beneficial and a variety of clinical and non-clinical group programs exist. Professionals (physicians, dietitians, behavioral therapists, nurses, etc.) and non-professionals lead some groups. Maintaining a lower body weight is a challenge since 90-95% of persons who lose weight subsequently regain it. Often after 6 months of weight loss treatment, the rate of weight loss usually decreases and a patient's weight tends to plateau. Long-term monitoring and support together with continuation of the combined modalities of dietary therapy, physical activity, and behavior therapy can help to maintain weight loss.

CHARACTERISTICS OF PATIENT

Patient

a. often skip meals
b. complains of feeling hungry after eating

Dietary Intervention

a. plan regular meal times
b. eat slowly
c. modify macronutrient content of meals to help with satiety

Patient

a. dines out frequently due to busy lifestyle
b. does not like to cook

Dietary Intervention

a. educate patient on more appropriate food choices when eating out
b. discuss balancing healthy food choices throughout the day
c. provide resources for preparing healthy meals for a hurried life

Patient

a. Eats fat-free foods but not losing weight
b. Reports eating small portions but not losing weight

Dietary Intervention

a. educate patient on the calorie content of fat-free foods
b. educate patient on nutrient density
c. measure portions

Patient

a. drinks coffee all day
b. eats one big meal

Dietary Intervention

a. educate patient that this can lead to increased body fat
b. educate patient about eating small regular meals

Chapter 7

READING NUTRITION LABELS

It is important to educate patients about reading nutrition labels. This guide will help them shop for foods that are nutritious and lower in Calories and fat to achieve weight loss.

The labels provide the following information:

1. Serving size
2. Servings per container
3. Calories per serving
4. Total fat per serving
5. Saturated fat per serving
6. Cholesterol content
7. Sodium content
8. Total carbohydrates
    a. Dietary fiber
    b. Sugars
9. Protein
10. Vitamin A
11. Vitamin C
12. Calcium
13. Iron
14. Percent daily

Following are some words frequently used in labels:

1. Calorie-free – less than 5 Calories per serving
2. Light (lite) – one-third less Calories or half the fat of the high-Calorie food or high fat food, or half the sodium of high sodium food
3. Fat-free – less than 0.5 grams of fat per serving
4. Low fat – 3 grams of fat per serving
5. Reduced or low fat – 25% less fat
6. Lean – less than 10 grams of fat, 4 grams of saturated fat and

95 mg of cholesterol per serving
7. Cholesterol-free – less than 2 grams of cholesterol and less than 2 grams of saturated fat per serving
8. Low Cholesterol – less than 20 mg of cholesterol and 2 grams of saturated fat per serving
9. Sugar-free – less than 0.5 grams of sugar per serving
10. High fiber – 5 grams or more of fiber per serving
11. Sodium-free – less than 5 mg of sodium per serving and no sodium chloride in the product
12. Very low sodium – 35 mg or less of sodium per serving
13. Low sodium – 140 mg of less of sodium per serving
14. Reduced or less sodium – 25% less sodium than the original amount in product

In addition to reading labels, it is also important to read ingredients. Ingredients in the greatest amount are listed first, and ingredients in the least amount are listed last. Reading the ingredients will help you avoid getting too much fat or sodium. Sources of fat and cholesterol in packaged foods are as follows:

1. Animal fat
2. Bacon fat
3. Butter
4. Chicken fat
5. Lard
6. Lamb fat
7. Pork fat
8. Turkey fat
9. Hardened fat
10. Beef fat
11. Ham fat
12. Egg and egg yolk solids

Transfatty Acids

Under the new regulations, by January 1, 2006, labels will have to include a new line for transfats, located directly under the line for saturated fat. This is the first major change in labeling requirements in a decade.

Nutrition Labeling

Product:	Check For:

Nutrition Facts
Serving Size 1 cup (228 g)
Servings Per Container 2

- Serving Size
- Number of Servings

Amount Per Serving
Calories 250 Calories from Fat 110

	% Daily Value*
Total Fat 12 g	18%
Saturated Fat 3 g	15%
Cholesterol 30 mg	10%
Sodium 470 mg	20%
Total Carbohydrate 31 g	10%
Dietary Fiber 0g	0%
Sugars 5g	
Protein 5g	

- Calories
- Total fat in grams
- Saturated fat
- Cholesterol
- Sodium

Here, the label gives the amounts for the different nutrients in one serving. This helps one to keep tract of how many calories and how many calories and how much fat, saturated fat, cholesterol, and sodium one is getting from different foods.

The "% Daily Value" shows how much of the recommended amounts the food provides in one serving, if you eat 2,000 calories a day. For example, one serving of this food gives you 18 percent of your total fat recommendation.

Vitamin A 4% • Vitamin C 2%
Calcium 20% • Iron 4%

*Percent Daily Values are based on a 2,000 calorie diet. Your daily values may be higher or lower depending on your Calorie needs.

	Calories	2,000	2,500
Total Fat	Less than	65g	80g
Sat Fat	Less than	20g	25g
Cholesterol	Less than	300mg	300mg
Sodium	Less than	2,400mg	2,400mg
Total Carbohydrate		300g	375g
Dietary Fiber		25g	30g

Calories per gram:
Fat 9 • Carbohydrates 4 • Protein 4

This is the recommended daily amount for each nutrient for two-calorie levels. If one eats a 2,000 calorie diet, one should be eating less than 65 grams of fat and less than 20 grams of saturated fat. If one eats 2,500 calories a day, one should eat less than 80 grams of fat and 25 grams of saturated fat. Daily amounts may be higher or lower, depending on the calories one eats.

Mounting scientific evidence shows that consumption of transfat, along with saturated fat and cholesterol, raises LDL cholesterol levels, and thereby increases the risk of .

The Food and Drug Administration estimates that the changes will save between $900 million and $1.8 million each year in medical costs, lost productivity, and pain and suffering.

Transfats develop during the process of hydrogenation, in which hydrogen is added to vegetable oil in order to turn the oil into a more solid fat. It's often found along with saturated fat in such foods as vegetable shortening, some margarines, crackers, candies, cookies, and fried and other processed foods.

But right now, there are no specific recommendations for transfat intake. Actual dietary intake of transfat is running at 1.5 to 2 percent of total calories, while intake of saturated fat is running at about 12 to 14 percent of calories. The combined total intake of trans and saturated fats should probably be under 10 percent.

The idea of the new labeling information is to help consumers make more informed and healthier choices. Whether this will actually happen is another question.

Manufacturers of dietary supplements will also be required to list transfat content, as well as saturated fat and cholesterol on the "Supplement Facts" panel when their products (such as nutrition and energy bars) contain more than trace amounts (0.5 grams).

The Food and Drug Administration (www.fda.gov) has more information on transfats, as does the American Dietetic Association (www.eatright.org).

Chapter 8

EATING OUT

People are eating out more frequently. Americans are spending about 43 percent of their food dollars on foods purchased away from home. People eat out either for necessity or pleasure. Eating out frequently means that an individual's diet will be high in fat, cholesterol and sodium. Even though many restaurants have started offering low fat dishes, one must be very careful making choices. Some of the concerns about eating out frequently are as follows:

1. Fats. High fat ingredients include cheese, butter or oil and the fat is all the more harmful when dishes are deep-fried or sautéed.

2. Portions. Portion sizes are very large. One is tempted to overeat.

3. Sodium content is high. This may be due to the use of excessive salt, or the use of ingredients that are high in sodium.

4. Fiber-rich foods are not used. Instead, meat and poultry are featured while fiber-rich foods are used as side dishes.

5. Beverage intake tends to be high, especially beer, wine, hard liquor or carbonated beverages.

STRATEGIES FOR EATING OUT

Keep hunger under control

- Don't skip a meal on the day you're going out to eat.
- Consider eating a light snack an hour or so before the meal to avoid overeating at the restaurant
- Choose a restaurant that offers a variety of foods, with low-fat options.
- Call the restaurant ahead of time, ask about healthy menu items.

Order more plant-based foods

- Treat yourself to your favorite vegetables, but don't smother them in high-fat dressings or rich creams.
- Order items that include whole-grain foods to get your fiber.
- Order fruits, vegetables and whole-grain foods. They are naturally low in calories and fat, and they'll fill you up with fiber and other health-enhancing nutrients.
- Fruits: pick salads and desserts that emphasize fruits, including apples, bananas, blueberries, grapefruit, grapes, kiwi, oranges, papaya, peaches, pears, pineapple, strawberries.
- Vegetables: pick salads, side and main dishes that include plenty of broccoli, carrots, cauliflower, cucumbers, green beans, bell peppers, dark leafy greens, mushrooms, spinach, tomatoes.
- Whole grains: pick entrees and sides that include whole-grain pasta, bread, rice, cereal.

Limit Fat

- Order baked, grilled.
- Ask for smaller portions of fatty foods – such as meats and fatty sauces – or ask for substitutions.

Cut back on condiments

- Taste your food before adding salt, butter, sauces and dressings.
- Order sauces and dressings on the side – small amounts add up!
- Substitute healthier condiments. For example, use mustard instead of mayonnaise, or pepper or lemon juice instead of salt.

Buffet eating

- Don't get tempted overfilling your plate. Choose healthier options.
- Make salad your first course, with plenty of veggies, fruit, and no-fat or low-fat dressing. Then go back for the entrée – or just eat more salad.

Mind your manners – it will help you

- Eat slowly. You will feel full faster.
- Chew thoroughly.
- Order food that requires work and slows your eating.
- Share your meal with a companion.

Order beverages with no or low calories

- Order water, sparkling water or mineral water with a twist of lemon – it's healthy, filling, and has no calories.
- For a hot drink, try black decaf coffee or black or green tea, minus sugar or other extras.

Wait before ordering dessert

- Finish the main dish. By the time you're done, you may not even want dessert.
- If you do order dessert, split it with a friend or take half of it home.

Leave food on your plate or ask for a doggie bag

- If you're tempted to clean your plate, ask your server to remove it.
- Take a doggie bag.

Effective in 1997, the Food and Drug Administration (FDA) began regulating nutrition and health claims on restaurant menus. Restaurants must provide nutrition information to back up nutrient and health claims. This applies to any type of eating establishment – from fast-food to four-star restaurants.

- Nutrient claims. These claims describe the amount of a nutrient in a food. For example, if a restaurant labels a selection as low-fat, it must be able to back up this claim and tell you how much fat is in a serving. Also ask about serving size. A server might tell you that a low-fat item has no more than 3 grams of fat per serving – but if the portions are twice the size of a standard serving, you're getting twice the fat.
- Health claims. These are claims about the link between a nutrient or food and a disease or health condition. For example, when a menu item has a heart symbol next to it and is called heart-heathy, it means that the item is low in fat, saturated fat and cholesterol. A diet low in saturated fat and cholesterol can lower your risk of heart disease.

Menu items described as healthy must be low in fat and saturated fat, and they can't be high in cholesterol or sodium. But there are no restrictions on calories. If you have questions about a nutrient or health claim on the menu, ask your server for more information.

FDA regulations for restaurant menus are more liberal than food labeling requirements. Restaurants do not have to:

- Provide full nutrition information for all menu selections.
- Provide full nutrition information for menu items that make nutrient or health claims – they just have to be able to back up the specific nutrient or health claim, either verbally or in writing.
- Confirm nutrient levels by laboratory analysis – they may use nutrient databases or cookbooks, so their calculations are less than scientific.

Restaurant dining guide

- Appetizer. Choose appetizers with vegetables, fruits or fish. Tomato juice, fresh fruit compote and shrimp cocktail served with lemon are good choices.
- Soup. The best choices are broth-based or tomato-based, such as consommé, gazpacho (a soup made of chopped raw vegetables, served cold), mulligatawny (chicken stock-based soup with curry) or minestrone (if cheese is not added). Creamed soups, chowders, pureed soups and, occasionally, fruit soups can contain heavy cream or egg yolks. Ask to be sure.
- Salad. Order lettuce or spinach salad with dressing on the side, preferably a low-fat version. Caesar, Greek and taco salads are higher in fat and calories. Chef salads are usually high in fat, cholesterol and calories because of cheese, eggs and meat.
- Bread. If you're offered a breadbasket, take one piece and ask your server to remove the basket. Choose whole grain bread, rolls, breadsticks, crackers or bagels. Muffins, garlic toast and croissants have more calories and fat.
- Side dish. Choose a baked potato, boiled new potatoes, steamed vegetables or rice, or fresh fruits instead of french fries, potato chips, onion rings or mayonnaise-based salads. Ask that no fat be used to prepare the vegetables or rice.
- Entrée. Look for descriptions that indicate lower fat, such as London broil, grilled chicken breast, lemon-baked fish, or broiled beef shish kebabs. Avoid items with high-fat descriptors, such as prime rib of beef, veal parmigiana, stuffed shrimp, fried chicken, fettuccine Alfredo, filet mignon with béarnaise sauce, shrimp tempura or fried rice. Choose pasta primavera or linguine with red tomato or clam sauce. Skip pasta with meat or cheese stuffing, or sauces that contain bacon, butter, cream or eggs.

Cooking terms	
Choose	**Avoid**
Baked Broiled (without added butter) Grilled Poached Roasted Steamed Sautéed or stir-fried in a small amount of oil, broth or water	A la king Au gratin Basted Breaded Buttered Broasted Sautéed or stir-fried in heavy oil Creamed Fricasseed Fried

Hidden sodium

- Au jus or in broth (although the terms can mean the food is served with juices obtained from cooking, many restaurants use a high-sodium, commercial meat base.)
- In cocktail sauce
- In tomato base
- Pickled
- Smoked
- Teriyaki

Chapter 9

POPULAR DIETS

Weight loss is a major concern for the Americans. Most surveys show that most Americans are trying to lose weight. Most people who are trying to lose weight are not using low Calorie diet and are not increasing their physical activity. Many try different popular diets. These diets usually appear in lay publications as opposed to medical and scientific literature. Many of these diet books contain half-truths and misinterpretation of biochemistry and physiology. Summary of some of the popular diets is given below.

I. LOW-CARBOHYDRATE, HIGH PROTEIN DIETS

A. The Zone Diet (Low Carbohydrate Diet) by Barry Sears, PhD. The basic premise of the diet is to balance between good and bad eicosanoids and the production of insulin. This book states that high carbohydrates consumption causes increased production of insulin, which in turn leads to obesity. The diet recommends 30% protein, 30% fat and 40% carbohydrate. This compares to the Dietary Guidelines that recommends 10-15% protein, less than 30% fat, and 55-60% carbohydrates, mainly from complex carbohydrates. This diet is also recommended for athletes.

There is little data that eicosanoids are responsible for diseases or the disease risk can be altered by changing eiconasids in the diet. People lose weight on this diet because it is low in total Calories. This diet cannot be sustained for a long time.

B. Adkins' (Very Low Carbohydrate Diet) New Diet Revolution, by Robert C Atkins, MD. The rationale for this diet is that carbohydrates intake promotes insulin secretion, which leads to weight gain. The difference with the zone diet is that Atkins diet recommends an extreme degree of carbohydrate restriction, to maintain ketosis (20–90gm/dl). Most grains, beans and vegetables are not allowed in the diet except for salad and some vegetables. Allowed foods are meat, butter and cream. Dr. Atkins claims that dietary ketosis depresses appetite and allows the body to burn its own fat.

There are many risks associated with this diet. Ketosis is not a natural state and we do not have the data for the long-term effects of this diet. This diet eliminates complex carbohydrates such as fruits and breads. This diet is high in saturated fat, protein and low in fiber. High protein diets can cause an excess of urate production due to the high purine content, which can lead to gout. Atkins' diet can produce short term weight loss but would be difficult to maintain for long time without any health risk.

C. **The South Beach Diet (Good/Bad Carbs)**
The rationale for this diet is to steer off high glycemic index foods, like white bread and beer, which raise blood sugar levels too quickly. During the first two weeks, fruits, bread, sugar, snacks, potatoes, pasta or rice are not allowed. Avoiding high-glycemic index foods eliminates insulin resistance and promotes weight loss. These claims haven not been scientifically proven, but at least this diet includes whole grains and fruits. Cut back on saturated fats.

D. **The "Sugar Busters" Diet by A. Leighton Steward.** This diet is based on the premise that high sugar foods contain high glycemic index (carrots, corn, beets, white potatoes, pasta, and bread) and the consumption of these foods lead to obesity. Authors state that high sugar diets cause increased insulin secretion, which in turn causes obesity.

This diet is not particularly dangerous to health, except for the fact it eliminates many vegetables that have nutritional value.

II. HIGH CARBOHYDRATES, LOW FAT DIETS

A. Life Choice Diet by Dean Ornish, MD. This is a very low fat diet (15-25 gm/day). The focus is on legumes, fruits, vegetables, and whole grains, processed foods and nonfat dairy products are eaten in moderation. The claims of this diet are based on scientific research. Results showed regression of coronary atherosclerosis in these patients who were maintained on low fat vegetarian diet, exercise and stress management. The American Heart Association has issued an advisory about using this diet for a long time. Their concerns were about a short-term increase in triglyceride and decrease in HDL cholesterol levels.

B. The New Pritkin Diet by Robert Pritkin. This diet is high in complex carbohydrates, moderate in protein, and very low in fat and consists of 5-6 meals per day.

This diet is too rigid and may be hard to sustain for a long time.

III. OTHER POPULAR DIETS

A. Emotional Eating

Dr. Phil's approach to weight loss involves "getting real." He suggests curbing emotional eating, surrounding yourself with a supportive circle of friends and family, and exercising. Don't eat sugar or saturated fats. Don't skip meals or eat after 8 p.m. Don't let saboteurs jealously tell you, "You look too thin." The claim is if you change your thinking and your attitude – and eat "high yield" foods – you'll change your weight. The diet plan is essentially low-calorie and high-protein. Much of Dr. Phil's advice is sound, if over-simplified. But the supplements he promotes are of unproved effectiveness, and not all overweight people eat emotionally.

B. Counting Points

Weekly support-group meetings and weigh-ins, food journaling and the "points system" help you eat properly and stay motivated. Don't eat whatever you please, but every food has a point value based on its fiber, fat and calorie content, and your daily intake has to stay below your allotted maximum. Points-based eating allows for safe and gradual weight loss. If you exercise, you can tack on daily bonus points. Nutritionists like any plan that promotes portion control and substitutes low-fat, high-fiber foods for fatty ones.

According to the author, blood type O's should eat animal protein, little carbohydrate, and no wheat products. Blood type B's should eat red meat, fish and dairy, but no chicken, shellfish, or wheat. Blood type AB's should follow a combination of diets for blood type A and B. This diet is not practical for everyday.

C. Do It Your Way

The book doesn't lay out a strict plan but offers common-sense advice from "masters" who have lost 20 lbs. or more and kept the weight off for at least three years. There are no rules, but the masters favor low-fat eating, regular mealtimes, food journaling, realistic goals and exercise. You'll lose weight successfully if you do it your way. But diets that claim you can eat all you want and still lose weight – or depend on such unscientific treatments as body wraps, injections and fat-burning supplements – are probably unreliable. This gimmick-free book relies on the old rule: to lose weight, burn more calories than you consume.

D. Exercise using the pedometer

Use the pedometer that comes with the book to monitor steps taken per day. Don't make lifestyle changes you'll give up on: reduce food intake 25% and increase daily steps by 500 (five flights of stairs) every week for 12 weeks. Counting steps is a more effective way to lose weight than counting calories.

Chapter 10

ETHNIC AND FAST FOODS

CHINESE

Foods recommended in Chinese restaurants are: steamed or stir fried vegetables, meats cooked in hot and spicy tomato sauce or served on a sizzling platter. Chinese food is high in sodium unless you specifically request that you do not want MSG (Monosodium Glutamate) used in your dish. Specific dishes recommended in Chinese restaurants are as follows:

Appetizers
Steamed dumplings
Roast pork strips
Beef or chicken satay

Soups
Hot and sour
Wonton
Sizzling rice with chicken or shrimp

Chicken

Hunan spice chicken
Chicken with vegetables
Chicken chop suey
Chicken stir fried with
Chinese cabbage and
Other vegetables

Meats
Beef and broccoli
Twice cooked pork
Pork with cabbage,
green peppers and
other vegetables)
Roast Pork with vegetables

Seafood
Shrimp with tomato sauce
Shrimp with broccoli

Vegetables
Vegetarian delight
Spicy green beans
Broccoli & black
Mushroom

Rice
Steamed
White
Fried rice

Noodles
Roast pork low mein
Chicken low mein
Vegetable low mein

Desserts
Lychee nuts
Ripe apple crunch

Low Calorie, Fat and Cholesterol Chinese Meals

Low Calorie/ Low Fat Model Meal	**Hot-and sour soup** Quantity: 1 cup Exchanges: 1 vegetable, 1 fat **Yu Hsiang chicken** Quantity: 1 cup (split order) Exchanges: 2 meat; 1 fat; 1 vegetable **Shrimp with broccoli and mushrooms** Quantity: 1 cup Exchanges: 2 meat; 1 fat; 1 vegetable **Steamed white rice** Quantity: 2/3 cup Exchanges: 2 starches **Fortune cookie** (read fortune; skip cookie)

Estimated Nutrient Evaluation	Calories	615
	Fat	27g (39% of calories)
	Protein	41g (27% of calories)
	Carbohydrate	51g (34% of calories)
	Cholesterol	150mg
	Sodium^{+}	1300mg

Low Calorie/ Low Cholesterol Model Meal	**Beef with broccoli and black Mushrooms** Quantity: 1 cup (split order) **Vegetarian delight** Quantity: 1 ½ cup **Steamed white rice** Quantity: 2/3 cup **Lychee nuts** Quantity: 1/2 cup

Estimated Nutrient Evaluation	Calories	590
	Fat	25g (38% of calories)
	Protein	33g (22% of calories)
	Carbohydrate	59g (40% of calories)
	Cholesterol	52mg
	Sodium^{+}	915mg

High Calorie, Low Fat and Cholesterol Chinese Meal

Higher Calorie/Low Fat Model	**Peking raviolis**, steamed Quantity: 2 Exchanges: 1 starch; 1 meat; 1 fat; ½ vegetable **Moo shi shrimp** Quantity: 2 pancakes; 1 cup filling (split order) Exchanges: 1 starch; 2 meats;1 fat; 2 vegetables **Vegetable lo mein noodles** Quantity: 1 ½ cups (split order) Exchanges: 3 starch; 1 fat; 1 vegetable **Tsing Tsao beer** Quantity: 12 oz. Exchanges: 1 starch; 1 fat	
Estimated Nutrient Evaluation	Calories Fat Protein Carbohydrate Alcohol Cholesterol Sodium+	911 24g (24% of calories) 43g (19% of calories) 112g (49% of calories) 8% calories 134mg 1300mg
Higher Calorie/Low Cholesterol Model Meal	**Sizzling rice** and chicken soup Quantity: 1 cup **Velvet chicken** Quantity: *1* cup (split order) **Szechwan fresh fish fillets** Quantity: *1* cup **Vegetable-fried rice** Quantity: *1* cup **Pineapple** Quantity: 1/2 cup	
Estimated Nutrient Evaluation	Calories Fat Protein Carbohydrate Alcohol Cholesterol Sodium+	687 23g (30% of calories) 43g (25% of calories) 77g (45% of calories) 8% calories 110mg 1700mg

Low Sodium Chinese Meals

Low[*] Sodium Model Meal	**Peking raviolis,** steamed (use sweet sauce and mustard) Quantity: 2 **Sizzling sliced chicken** with vegetables Quantity: 1 cup (split order) **Beef chow mein** Quantity: 1 cup **Steamed white rice** Quantity: 1 cup	
Estimated Nutrient Evaluation	Calories	814
	Fat	33g (37% of calories)
	Protein	51g (25% of calories)
	Carbohydrate	77g (38% of calories)
	Cholesterol	135mg
	Sodium[+]	1200mg

[*] Requested that no MSG and less soy sauce be used.

[+] Sodium values are based on usually preparation methods determined from several Chinese cookbooks. If no MSG, less soy and less other sauces are requested, sodium intake can easily be lowered.

Terms of Chinese cuisine

- **Bean curd** - known as **'tofu'** to Americans, made from soy beans and formed into blocks, used sliced or cubed in soups or dishes.
- **Black bean sauce -** a thick, brown sauce made of fermented soy beans, salt, and wheat flour, frequently used in Cantonese cooking
- **Bok choy** - looks like a cross between celery and cabbage; also known as Chinese chard.
- **Hoisin sauce** - a sweet and spicy thick- sauce made from soy beans, sugar, garlic, chili, and vinegar.
- **Lily buds** - dried, golden-colored with a light flowery flavor; also called lotus buds and tiger lily buds; used in entrees and soups.
- **Lycee** - crimson-colored fruit with translucent flesh around a brown seed, closely resembling a white grape.
- **Monosodium glutamate** (MSG) - a white powder used in small amounts to bring out and enhance the flavors of ingredients.
- **Napa cabbage** - also referred to as Chinese cabbage, it has thick-ribbed crinkled leaves.

- **Oyster sauce** - a rich thick sauce made of oysters, their cooking liquid, and soy sauce; frequently used in Cantonese dishes.

FAST FOODS

Fast food places offer low-priced foods and quick service. Many fast food restaurants have started offering salad bars, baked potatoes, beans and sugar free soft drinks. Be cautious in choosing foods from fast food restaurants! Generally, fast foods are high in fat, saturated fat and sodium. The nutrient content of these foods is given in the Appendix section of this book. Recommended foods from the fast food restaurants are:

1. Plain hamburger with tomato, lettuce (no mayonnaise). Avoid the cheese, bacon and ham.
2. Grilled chicken sandwich
3. Chef salad with low fat dressing
4. Baked potato with chili and light cheese
5. Low fat frozen yogurt
6. Thin "n" crispy pizza
7. Grilled vegetarian pizza

Foods to Avoid in Fast Food Restaurants:

1. Fried Chicken
2. Croissant sandwiches
3. Biscuit sandwiches
4. Sauces
5. Bacon
6. Cheese sauce
7. Sour cream
8. Salad dressing (regular)
9. Breaded and fried foods
10. Fried desserts
11. Double and Triple Decker burgers

Low Calorie, Fat and Cholesterol Fast Food Meals

Low Calorie/ Low Fat Meal McDonald's	Cheeseburger Garden Salad with reduced-calorie French Dressing (1 Tbsp)

	Ice tea (unsweetened) Vanilla frozen yogurt cone	
Estimated Nutrient Evaluation	Calories Fat Protein Carbohydrate Cholesterol Sodium⁺	600 22g (32% of calories) 25g (16% of calories) 79g (52% of calories) 185mg 1500mg

Low Calorie/ Low Cholesterol Meal Hardee's	Chef Salad with reduced-calorie Italian dressing (2 Tbsp) Vanilla Shake	
Estimated Nutrient Evaluation	Calories Fat Protein Carbohydrate Cholesterol Sodium^{+}	628 24g (34% of calories) 34g (22% of calories) 69g (44% of calories) 70mg 1410mg

Higher Calorie/Low Cholesterol Meal Wendy's	Baked potato w/chili and cheese (request light on cheese) French dressing (2tbsp)	
Estimated Nutrient Evaluation	Calories Fat Protein Carbohydrate Cholesterol Sodium^{+}	770 30g (35% of calories) 28g (15% of calories) 97g (50% of calories) 45mg 1200mg

FAST FOODS

Low Calorie, Fat and Cholesterol Fast Food Meals

Low Calorie/ Low Fat Meal McDonald's	McGrilled chicken sandwich Garden Salad with lite Vinaigrette (1/2 package)

	Vanilla frozen yogurt cone	
Estimated Nutrient Evaluation	Calories	475
	Fat	9g (16% of calories)
	Protein	34g (28% of calories)
	Carbohydrate	68g (54% of calories)
	Cholesterol	190mg
	Sodium	775mg

Low Calorie/ Low Cholesterol Meal Boston Chicken	Chicken Soup Cornbread muffin Buttered corn Cucumber Salad	
Estimated Nutrient Evaluation	Calories	624
	Fat	24g (34% of calories)
	Protein	22g (14% of calories)
	Carbohydrate	82g (52% of calories)
	Cholesterol	61mg
	Sodium	1374mg

Higher Calorie/ Low Fat Meal Kenny Rogers	White Meat – 1/4 (remove skin and wing) Honey-baked beans Macaroni and cheese Corn muffin	
Estimated Nutrient Evaluation	Calories	609
	Fat	16g (16% of calories)
	Protein	34g (24% of calories)
	Carbohydrate	69g (45% of calories)
	Cholesterol	126mg
	Sodium	1676mg

High Calorie, Low Cholesterol Fast Foods

Higher calorie/Low Cholesterol Model Meal: Boston Chicken	Dark meat – 1/4 (skin removed) New potatoes Zucchini marinara Cornbread Fruit salad	
Estimated Nutrient Evaluation	Calories	757
	Fat	29g (35% of calories)
	Protein	37g (19% of calories)

	Carbohydrate	87g (46% of calories)
	Cholesterol	153mg
	Sodium	1517mg

Low Sodium Fast Food Meal

Low Sodium Model Meal: Kenny Rogers	Chicken noodle soup (small) Roasted chicken sandwich (request small amount of dressing) Cinnamon apples	
Estimated Nutrient Evaluation	Calories	665
	Fat	20g (27% of calories)
	Protein	43g (26% of calories)
	Carbohydrate	80g (47% of calories)
	Cholesterol	226mg
	Sodium	359mg

Pizza – High Fat Choices

High Fat Choices	extra cheese (all types) pepperoni sausage Anchovies Bacon Meatballs Prosciutto

RECOMMENDATIONS:

- Take the salad dressing on the side.
- Go light on the cheese.
- Substitute spicy chicken for the sausage (or pepperoni) on this pizza.
- Instead of the extra cheese, put on more onions and sliced tomatoes.
- Get pizza cheeseless.
- Wrap extra to take home.

Low Calorie, Low Fat, Low Cholesterol Pizza and Salad

Low Calorie/ Low Fat Meal Godfather's	Garden Salad with Italian dressing, reduced calorie, 2 tbs Original cheese pizza, 2 slices

Estimated Nutrient Evaluation	Calories	582
	Fat	18g (28% of calories)
	Protein	22g (15% of calories)
	Carbohydrate	83g (57% of calories)
	Cholesterol	44mg
	Sodium	1037mg

Low Calorie/ Low Cholesterol Meal Little Caesar's Pizza	Greek salad with Italian dressing, with extra vinegar Pan! Vegetable pizza 2 slices	
Estimated Nutrient Evaluation	Calories	540
	Fat	24g (40% of calories)
	Carbohydrate	56g (42% of calories)
	Cholesterol	43mg
	Sodium	1387mg

High Calorie, Low Fat, Low Cholesterol Pizza and Salad

Higher Calorie/Low Fat Meal Domino's	Veggie pizza, hand tossed 4 slices	
Estimated Nutrient Evaluation	Calories	836
	Fat	20g (22% of calories)
	Protein	60g (28% of calories)
	Carbohydrate	104g (50% of calories)
	Cholesterol	76mg
	Sodium	2050mg

Higher Calorie/Low Cholesterol Meal Pizza Hut	Tossed salad, 2 cups from salad bar (all vegetables) with Ranch dressing, 2 tbsp with vinegar Veggie Lovers Pizza 2 slices

Estimated Nutrient Evaluation	Calories	621
	Fat	25g (36% of calories)
	Protein	28g (18% of calories)
	Carbohydrate	71g (46% of calories)
	Cholesterol	44mg
	Sodium	1003mg

Low Sodium Pizza and Salad

Low Sodium Meal California Pizza Kitchen's Grilled	Field greens salad, ½ order with Balsamic Dijon Vinaigrette, 1 tbsp, with extra balsamic vinegar Eggplant Cheese less pizza, 3 slices	
Estimated Nutrient Evaluation	Calories	593
	Fat	17g (25% of calories)
	Protein	26g (18% of calories)
	Carbohydrate	0g (57% of calories)
	Cholesterol	0mg
	Sodium	1850mg

MEXICAN FOOD

The fat content of Mexican foods is very high. Popular foods include nachos with guacamole, cheese and sour cream, tacos, cheese enchiladas and refried beans. Healthy choices are soft chicken tacos, chicken or beef fajitas. Some Mexican restaurants have started offering "Border Lights". These foods include chicken tacos, taco salad, bean and beef burritos, and these are all excellent choices because they contain half the fat of the regular menu. Recommended Mexican foods are as follows:

1. Tostado with hot salsa
2. Black bean soup
3. Chili con carne
4. Gazpacho
5. Mexican salad
6. Taco salad
7. Fajitas
8. Enchiladas
9. Burritos
10. Tostadas
11. Chiliverde
12. MolePollo
13. AnozconPollo
14. Mexican Rice
15. Black bean
16. Tortillas (Flour or corn)
17. Flan

Low Calorie, Low Fat Mexican Meal

Low Calorie Low Fat Meal	Chili con carne Dinner Salad (hold cheese and dressing; order salsa) Quantity: 2 cups, Salsa for dressing Chicken taco, soft Quantity: 1	
Estimated Nutrient Evaluation	Calories Fat Protein Carbohydrate Cholesterol Sodium	480 19g (35% of calories) 31g (26% of calories) 47g (39% of calories) 67mg 1600mg

High Calorie, Low Fat and Low Cholesterol Mexican Meal

Higher Calorie/Low Fat Meal	Black bean soup Quantity: 1 cup Chili verde served with 2 flour tortillas Quantity: 1 ½ cups Mexican rice, Quantity: 1/3 cup Refried beans, Quantity: 1/3 cup Mexican beer, Quantity: 12 oz	
Estimated Nutrient Evaluation	Calories Fat Protein Carbohydrate Alcohol Cholesterol Sodium	992 30g (27% of calories) 42g (17% of calories) 119g (48% of calories) 8% calories 96mg 2100mg
Higher Calorie/Low Cholesterol Meal	Tostado chips Quantity: 10 Salsa Quantity: 2 tbsp Burrito, bean and cheese (request extra lettuce and diced tomatoes, 1 cup) Quantity: 1 Chicken enchilada (hold cheese) Quantity: 1 Mexican Rice Quantity: 1/3 cup Black beans (request substitute for refried beans) Quantity: 1/3 cup	

Estimated Nutrient Evaluation	Calories Fat Protein Carbohydrate Cholesterol Sodium	780 29g (35% of calories) 37g (19% of calories) 92g (47% of calories) 60mg 2000mg

Low Sodium Mexican Meal

Low Sodium Meal	Mexican salad with shredded, spicy chicken, black beans, lettuce, tomatoes, and onion Quantity: 3—4 cups Guacamole (on the side; hold sour cream) Quantity: ¼ cup Salsa verde for dressing Quantity: 4 tbsp Corn tortillas Quantity: 2 Flan (split order)	
Estimated Nutrient Evaluation	Calories Fat Protein Carbohydrate Cholesterol Sodium	720 25g (31% of calories) 50g (28% of calories) 70g (39% of calories) 197mg (12% from Flan) 9500mg

Terms of Mexican Cuisine

- **Arroz** - Spanish word for rice, Mexican rice is made from long-grain white rice with sautéed tomatoes, onion, and garlic added for flavor.
- **Burrito** - a wheat flour tortilla (soft, not fried) filled with chicken, beef, or cheese in addition to refried beans; served rolled up and covered with a light tomato-based enchilada sauce.
- **Carne** - Spanish word for meat.
- **Cerveza** - Spanish word for beer.
- **Ceviche** - raw fish soaked or "cooked" in lime or lemon juice for many hours and served as an appetizer or light meal.
- **Chalupa** -"little boat," a one-dish meal of corn meal topped with meat or chicken beans and cheese.

- **Chili** - there are over 100 different types of chilies native to Mexico. They are of different shapes, sizes, and colors, and they vary in level of spiciness from mild to hot, hotter, and hottest. Chilies are available fresh or dried.
- **Chili** con carne - usually simply called "chili" is a thick soup made with tomatoes, onions, peppers, beans, and ground or shredded beef; often served with raw chopped onions and shredded cheese.
- **Chimichanga** - flour tortilla filled with beef, chicken, cheese, and/or beans; deep fried and served topped with tomato-based sauce.
- **Chorizo** - Mexican pork sausage, hot and highly seasoned.
- **Cilantro** - leafy green herb with a strong flavor frequently used in Mexican cooking; also called coriander.
- **Enchiladas** - corn tortillas dipped in enchilada sauce, lightly fried, and then filled with a choice of chicken, beef, or cheese and served topped with light tomato-based enchilada sauce.

ITALIAN

Low Calorie, Low Fat, Italian Meal

Low Calorie Low Fat Meal	Arugula and Belgian endive salad (request balsamic vinegar on the side) Quantity: 2 cups Fusilli (request marinara or tomato sauce to top) Quantity: 2 starch Shrimp primavera (eat half) Quantity: 1 ½ cups	
Estimated Nutrient Evaluation	Calories	450
	Fat	11g (21% of calories)
	Protein	38g (34% of calories)
	Carbohydrate	51g (45% of calories)
	Cholesterol	160mg
	Sodium	650mg
Low Calorie Low Fat Model Meal	Marinated mushrooms Quantity: 1 cup Ziti Bolognese Quantity: 1 ½ cups Parmesan cheese for above Quantity: 1 tbsp	

	Coffee Quantity: 1 cup or more	
Estimated Nutrient Evaluation	Calories Fat Protein Carbohydrate Cholesterol Sodium	550 20g (32% of calories) 28g (21% of calories) 65g (47% of calories) 55mg 1100mg
Higher Calorie/Low Fat Meal	(split entire meal, portions shown are already divided) Italian bread Quantity: 2 small pieces, hold butter or oil Marinated vegetables (carrots, cauliflower, broccoli florets, Italian green beans) Quantity: 1 cup Angel hair pasta with white clam sauce Quantity: 1 ½ cups Veal piccata Quantity: 4 ozs Fresh raspberries with Kirsch (hold whipped cream) Quantity: ½ cup	

High Calorie, Low Fat, Low Cholesterol Italian Meal

Estimated Nutrient Evaluation	Calories Fat Protein Carbohydrate Cholesterol Alcohol Sodium	937 34g (33% of calories) 49g (21% of calories) 90g (38% of calories) 140mg (38% of calories) 8% of calories 1180mg
Higher Calorie/Low Cholesterol Meal	Tortellini in broth Quantity: 1 cup Insalata di casa (dressing on the side) Quantity: 1 cup Basil vinaigrette dressing (on the side) Quantity: 1 tbsp Veal cacciatore Quantity: ½ portion (1/2 in doggie bag) Spaghetti (hold sauce and use that from entrée) Quantity: 1 ½ cups	

Estimated Nutrient Evaluation	Calories	870
	Fat	28g (29% of calories)
	Protein	48g (22% of calories)
	Carbohydrate	89g (41% of calories)
	Cholesterol	100mg
	Alcohol	8% of calories
	Sodium	1050mg

Low Sodium Italian Meals

Low Sodium Meal	**Clams steamed in white wine** Quantity: 10 clams (1/2 order) **Linguini** (request served without sauce) Quantity: 1 ½ cups (split order) **Chicken in wine sauce** (request limit additional salt) Quantity: 4 ozs. **Italian Ice** Quantity: 1 cup	
Estimated Nutrient Evaluation	Calories	810
	Fat	29g (32% of calories)
	Protein	30g (15% of calories)
	Carbohydrate	65g (47% of calories)
	Cholesterol	170mg
	Sodium	680mg

Pastas

Pasta, meaning "paste" or "dough" is a staple food item in Italian restaurants. Pasta is created from flour (sometimes all-purpose flour), water, and/or eggs. These ingredients create a wide variety of different pastas, from angel hair to ziti.

Unlike Italy, many differently colored and spiced pastas are served in American restaurants today. There are whole-wheat, tomato, spinach, and artichoke, to name a few. Some of these are listed below.

- **Agnolotti** - crescent-shaped pieces of pasta, stuffed with one ingredient or a combination of cheese, meat, and spinach.
- **Angel hair** - the thinnest and finest of the long" pasta family, it is quite light in consistency and often served with light sauces.

- **Cannelloni** - large, tubular pasta, similar to manicotti, it is stuffed with one ingredient or a combination of cheese, meat, and spinach.
- **Capellitti** - meaning a "little hat," these are small, stuffed pastas that look like little tortellini; often stuffed with cheese and meat.
- **Fettucini** - flat, long noodle about 1/4-inch wide (wider than linguine).
- **Fusilli** - spiral-shaped long pasta, fusilli is round like spaghetti.
- **Gnocchi** - little dumplings, in ½-inch pieces made from either flour, potato, or a combination of both; often topped with sauce.
- **Lasagne** - the widest noodle among the long, flat pasta; found with either smooth or scalloped edges.
- **Linguine** - flat, long noodle about 1/8-inch wide (thinner than fettucini).
- **Manicotti** - long, tubular noodle about 2 inches in diameter, most often stuffed with cheese and/or meat and served with tomato sauce.
- **Mostaccioli** - short, tubular noodle about 1 ½ inches long.
- **Penne** - short, tubular noodle quite similar to mostaccioli and rigatoni.
- **Polenta** - corn meal and water mixture, which is cooked, poured on a board to harden, and served with a sauce.
- **Ravioli** - pasta squares, with corrugated edges, stuffed with cheese, spinach, or meats in combination or singly.
- **Rigatoni** - short, tubular noodle quite similar to penne and mostaccioli.
- **Risotto** - Italian short-grain rice that has a creamy consistency when cooked; often mixed with butter and cheese before serving.
- **Shells** - noodles in the shape of conch shells, called conchiglie in Italian, and found in a variety of sizes sometimes larger ones are stuffed, and most are served topped with tomato sauce.
- **Spaghetti** - thin, round pasta known pasta (also called vermicelli) the most commonly know pasta in America.
- **Tortelini** - small pastas, stuffed and joined at the end to form a ring; a larger version of capellitti.
- **Ziti** - short, tubular pasta similar to mostacciooi.

Chapter 11

INCORPORATION OF WEIGHT MANAGEMENT PROGRAM IN PRIMARY CARE PRACTICE

Barriers to successful physician-delivered dietary counseling regarding weight reduction by physicians in the US have included lack of training in nutrition, lack of time, lack of support staff with nutrition training, and reimbursement concerns. Additional factors include: beliefs about the effectiveness of intervention, concerns about patient response and compliance, knowledge about risk factors and perceived unpalatableness of certain diets. Survey data have revealed that physicians who feel prepared and competent to offer dietary lifestyle counseling are more likely to be willing to intervene around dietary practices to provide dietary counseling to their patients. Although physicians are thought by many to be in an advantageous position to promote lifestyles modification to promote weight reduction, few physicians place emphasis on diet. Medical educators have felt that improving the nutrition education of physicians would increase the inclusion of nutrition in patient care. However, having the knowledge does not necessarily guarantee appropriate nutrition related patient care. Nutritionists have identified core competencies in nutrition that should be mastered by the medical practitioner. It is believed that some of the barriers to physician-delivered dietary intervention can be addressed with an effective and efficient educational program that builds counseling skills and incorporates the use of reminders and easily used dietary assessment tools.

ALGORITHM FOR PHYSICIAN-DELIVERED WEIGHT MANAGEMENT COUNSELING INTERVENTION

Advise lowering dietary fat	• Your BMI is high (explain BMI). Your dietary fat intake is high. High fat intake increases your risk of getting heart disease and cancer. We need to develop a plan to replace high fat food with foods that taste good but are low in fat.
Assess - **past experience** - **current diet**	• Have you ever tried to lower the amount of fat and cholesterol in your diet? What changes did you make? • What strategies helped?
Advise increasing fiber intake	• Your dietary record shows that your fiber intake is low. Lower fiber intake increases your risk of getting cancer. We need to develop a plan to increase fiber in your diet.
Assess - **past experience** - **current diet**	• Have you tried to increase the amount of fiber in your diet? What changes did you make? • What problems did you have making changes? What strategies helped?
Advise about alcohol intake	• Your alcohol intake is high. High alcohol intake increases your risk of getting cancer. What changes did you make?
Advise about physical activity	• Exercise is very important in order to lose weight. • Are you doing any exercise program now? • Set goals for exercise.
Develop plan - **ways to deal with expected problems** - **dietary fat intake goal** - **fiber intake goal** - **provide handouts**	• What problems would you expect in making these changes? • How do you think you can deal with them? • Negotiate dietary goals with patient. • Set realistic goals about how much weight the patient should lose. • Individualize the program.
Arrange follow-up contact	• Address concern.

ALGORITHM FOR INCORPORATING OVERWEIGHT/OBESITY PROGRAM DURING OFFICE VISIT

Since the physician is very busy, a flow chart below shows how the patient's visit can be used for screening overweight/obese patients during the regular office visit.

1. Patient check in → Receptionist
   (give Weight Readiness questionnaire)

2. Patient get → Nurse
   a. Height, Weight
   b. BMI
   c. WHR

3. If BMI > 25 → Nurse
   (make a notation for physician)

4. Patient → Physician

   a. Medical check up
   b. History
   c. Talk about factors and weight
   d. If time permits, give counseling intervention tips
   e. List handouts to be given by the nurse or the receptionist

5. Give handouts as indicated by physician → Receptionist/Nurse

6. Schedule return visit → Very important

COMPREHENSIVE TREATMENT MODEL FOR WEIGHT MANAGEMENT IN OVERWEIGHT AND OBESE PATIENTS IN PRIMARY CARE

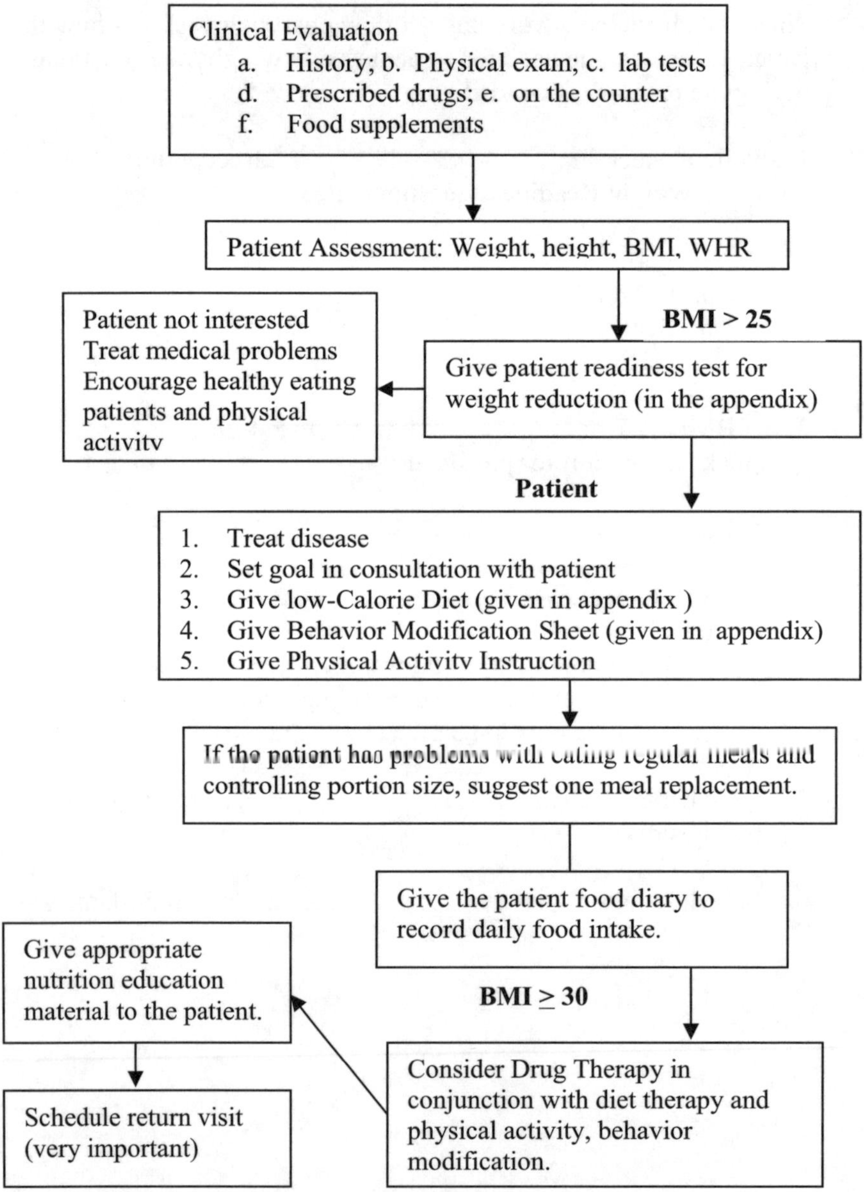

Chapter 12

HEALTHY WEIGHT 2010: OBJECTIVES FOR ACHIEVING AND MAINTAINING A HEALTHY POPULATION

Goals

The goals of the Healthy Weight 2010 objectives are to:

- Improve quality of life by reducing disease and disability associated with obesity.
- Increase quantity of life by reducing premature death associated with obesity.
- Reduce disparities and social stigma related to obesity.
- Promote healthy behaviors for weight control and weight management.
- Prevent weight gain that may lead to or exacerbate obesity and its co-morbidities.
- Educate the public of health risks associated with obesity and its co-morbidities.
- Increase access to appropriate medical evaluation and treatment of obesity.
- Improve health communication dealing with weight control between health professionals, managed care organizations and patients, and providers of weight control-related services and consumers.
- Form partnerships with organizations, businesses, and governmental health agencies (local, state, federal) to improve data collection and increase research funding with regard to obesity.

Review of Healthy People 2000 Objectives for Overweight

A Department of Health and Human Services (DHHS) progress report (June 1999) showed 20% of the Healthy People 200 objectives moving away from their targets, including the effort to reduce the prevalence of overweight in the US. From the hundreds of objectives in Healthy People 2000, only three directly addressed the issue of overweight.

Healthy People 2000 neglected to include overweight or obesity as a separate focus area. According to Surgeon General David Satcher, overweight or obesity is expected to be announced as a Leading Health Indicator for Healthy People 2010 at DHHS's conference, Partnerships for Health in the New Millennium: Launching Healthy People 2010, in January 2000. The progress report of Healthy People 2000 Objectives is given in Table 1.

Leading Health Indicators were developed to "be presented to the general public and non-health professionals as an introduction to Healthy People 2010." As recommended by the Institute of Medicine (IOM), leading health indicators will be followed closely over a 10-year period. AOA applauds the DHHA for taking an important step in recognizing obesity as a major public health problem that requires immediate attention to improve the health of the nation.

The DHHS acknowledges that with "the development of these indicators, it will be essential to identify a small set of measures that will better communicate with the general public and new partners such as managed care organizations and businesses." Establishing measurable objectives for overweight and obesity is critical for collecting data and monitoring progress.

The public must be thoroughly informed about obesity. They should know that obesity is difficult, but possible, to manage. Obesity does not occur overnight. It has a long duration and can frequently recur if not managed properly. It has a definite morbid process and affects the entire body. Understanding the causes and health risks of obesity, its assessment, prevention and treatment strategies, and the benefits of losing excess weight should become common public knowledge.

TABLE 1
Healthy People 2000 Objectives

Focus Area	Objectives #	Objective	*Progress Report
Physical Activity Nutrition Heart Disease and Stroke	1.2 2.3 15.10	 Reduce overweight prevalence	• The prevalence of overweight increased substantially among all groups between 1976-80 and 1994 • For all adults aged 20-74 the increase was 35 percent. • Similar increases were seen in the other demographics and age breakdowns.
Physical Activity Nutrition	1.7 2.7	Increased sound weight loss practices.	• Sound weight loss practice among overweight people, aged 12 years and over, continued to decline throughout the 1990's in all subgroups except overweight Hispanic women (the lowest subgroup in 1991). • The proportion of self-reported overweight adults who report consuming fewer calories, and exercising more, decreased from 1985-1995.
Nutrition	2.20		• The proportion of worksites with 50 or more employees that offer programs for employees increased from 17 percent in 1985 to 31 percent in 1992. • AOA note: while the

			progress report shows improvement, the 1995 baseline data for this objective for the year 2010, indicates that 14 percent of worksites offered weight management groups, classes, workshops, or lectures. This indicates a setback from the significant improvement shown in 1992 as well as from the original data in 1985.

**Progress toward Year 2000 Objectives as reported in Healthy People 2010: Draft for Public Comment.*

Objectives for Increasing Public Understanding of Obesity

Number	Objective
1	Health risks of overweight and obesity
2	Body Mass Index (BMI)
3	Multi-factorial components of causation of obesity
4	Benefits of weight loss
5	Treatment options for obesity
6	Setting reasonable weight goals
7	Maternal obesity and risk to infant

Medications for treating children with obesity have not yet been thoroughly studied or approved, but there is hope that pharmacotherapy will allow for safe and effective treatment of the most severe cases of childhood obesity. The increase in pharmacotherapy to treat obesity-related diseases in children, such as diabetes and hypertension, has created the need to investigate the benefits of attacking the primary problem of obesity with medication.

Approximately 25% of children and adolescents are overweight, a figure which has doubled in 30 years. Diabetes, hypertension and other obesity-related chronic diseases, prevalent among adults, are now becoming more common among youth. Excess weight during childhood and adolescence has been found to predict overweight for adults. This trend, along with prevalence data for youth and adults, suggests that quality and quantity of life are compromised if obesity is not contained.

Persons with obesity are at risk of developing one or more serious medical conditions. Obesity is associated with more than 30 medical conditions. Strong relationships have been scientifically established between obesity and at least 15 conditions, including arthritis, breast cancer, heart disease, colorectal cancer, type 2 diabetes, endometrial cancer, end-stage renal disease, gallbladder disease, hypertension, liver disease, low back pain, renal cell cancer, obstructive sleep apnea, stroke, and urinary incontinence. Evidence continues to mount linking obesity and several other diseases, disorders, conditions, and complications.

Poor diet and inactivity, contributors of obesity, are responsible for between 300,000 and 587,000 deaths a year, making it the second leading cause of preventable death in the US Lifelong management of obesity, using strategies such a lifestyle changes in diet and physical activity, drug therapy and surgery, is essential to improving health, maintaining an improved health status for a longer time, reducing absenteeism in the workplace, and reducing healthcare costs.

Objectives for Improving Weight Status

Number	Objective
1	Stabilizing weight
2	Achieving and maintaining healthy weight
3	Prevalence of healthy weight
4	Obesity prevalence in adults
5	Overweight prevalence in adults
6	Obesity prevalence in children and adolescents
7	Physical Activity for adult weight control
8	Physical Activity for weight control in children
9	Nutrition for adult weight control
10	Nutrition for weight control in children
11	Compliance of recommendations for maternal weight gain
12	Obesity as a risk factor for diseases
13	Absenteeism in the workplace due to obesity

Implementing Obesity Education Programs

Educating the public on the causes, prevention and treatment methods, and health risks of overweight and obesity, is critical to reversing the obesity epidemic. Population specific programs and messages should be culturally and linguistically appropriate to effectively translate information on obesity. Health professionals must be properly trained to follow an on-going process of evaluating, preventing, treating and managing overweight and obesity in their patients.

The public health community agrees to the need for obesity education, yet little progress has been made in implementing the concept. Schools, worksites, doctor's offices, managed care settings, and communities (health departments, social clubs and faith-based groups) are instrumental units for disseminating messages about obesity. Individuals, families, and communities must be mobilized to respond to the obesity epidemic.

Patient education is necessary to adequately control and prevent adverse health outcomes from chronic diseases. Research on hypertension and diabetes education, both of which are associated with obesity, indicates that even patients who have attended formal education programs failed to know the basics of their disease and self-management skills.

Obesity requires appropriate and sufficient education for patients of all literacy levels. Achieving success in patient communication requires appropriate written materials, oral communication, and visual presentation. Patient education needs ingenuity and commitment of necessary resources.

Practical education programs, modeled after successful campaigns which as the National Cholesterol Education Program could raise awareness of the importance of healthy body weight to health.

Objectives for Implementing Obesity Education Programs

Number	Objective
1	Elementary, secondary, and undergraduate healthy weight programs
2	Educating parents about children's healthy weight

3	Worksite weight management program availability
4	Worksite weight management program participation
5	Counseling and screening on obesity
6	Managed care and access to weight management programs
7	Healthy weight programs in communities
8	Reducing disparities through obesity education
9	Obesity education for primary care physicians
10	Smoking cessation & weight management programs
11	Worksite back injury prevention & weight management programs
12	Obesity, body image and eating disorder behaviors

Integrating Obesity Management into the Public Health Infrastructure

The impact of obesity is manifest not only on the nation's health, but also on the nation's economy. The high economic cost of obesity is a clear contributor to today's growing health care costs. Obesity has increased direct costs, due to greater use of medical services, and indirect costs, due to reduced productivity stemming from related illnesses and premature death.

Current, indirect strategies to control the incidence and prevalence of overweight and obesity, and its co-morbidities, have failed. Communities are in search of new initiatives that directly address the problem of obesity. New strategies for managing obesity must be integrated into the public health infrastructure, which includes community development. Constructing and properly maintaining sidewalks, parks and recreation areas, and securing safe streets for walking to schools and stores, can help to promote healthy lifestyles in communities.

Obtaining health insurance is often difficult for individuals with obesity, who are frequently denied access due to their weight. When they do obtain insurance, most insurance plans fail to offer reimbursement for weight loss or weight maintenance services, including surgery and pharmacy benefits.

More research is needed to determine effective strategies in preventing obesity, and the scientific data must be translated into a usable measure that can be tracked for progress. Strategies, however, must be put into effect immediately while research is planned and conducted.

Establishing lines of communication between traditional health partnerships and non-traditional partnerships, in which public health extends to areas such as transportation, urban planning and environmental planning, is an important step toward developing communities able to manage the problem of obesity.

Objectives for Integrating Obesity Management into the Public Health Infrastructure

Number	Objective
1	City planning for healthy weight communities
2	Access to health insurance for obesity
3	Measurement of obesity in data collection
4	Health communication regarding obesity

Source: *American Obesity Association*

Chapter 13

Summary

OVERWEIGHT OBESITY TREATMENT

I. Patient Evaluation
   A. Medical examination
   B. Prescription Drugs
   C. Over the counter drugs
   D. Food supplements
   E. Weight, height, BMI, WHR
   F. Patient Readiness Test for losing weight

II. Diet Therapy
   A. 24 hour recall, or food intake record
   B. Previous history of weight reduction diets
   C. Determine patient's food likes and dislikes and allergies
   D. Low Calorie Diet – 1200 Calories for Women and 1400 Calories for Men
   E. Individualize Diet Instructions

III. Behavior Modification
   A. Life style questions
   B. One large meal eater vs. snackers
   C. Binge Eating
   D. Sweet Tooth
   E. Give list of behavior modification tips emphasizing if there are any of the above or other problems

IV. Physical Activity
   A. Assess present physical activity
   B. Based on medical conditions and present physical activity, prescribe appropriate physical activity

V. Meal Replacement. One meal replacement may be recommended for those patients who are unable to eat 3 meals or have problems with controlling portion size.

VI. Drug Therapy. Drug therapy may be considered for patients who have BMI > 30 and/or who have been unsuccessful with traditional weight reduction diets. This must be done in conjunction with diet therapy, behavior modification and physical activity.

VII. Combination Therapy
  A. Diet Therapy and Behavior Modification
  B. Diet Therapy + Behavior Modification + Physical Activity
  C. Diet Therapy + Behavior Modification + Physical Activity + Drug Therapy
  D. Diet Therapy + Behavior Modification + Physical Activity + one Common Meal Replacement (e.g., Slim Fast, Boost, Ensure)
  E. Diet Therapy + Behavior Modification + Physical Therapy + Drug Therapy + one Meal Replacement

VIII. Patient Education
  A. Reading Nutrition Labeling
  B. Tips on eating out
  C. Skipping Meals
  D. Binge Eating
  E. Physical Activity

IX. Diet and Lifestyle Changes
  A. **Avoid Trans-Fatty Acids and Partly Hydrogenated Fats ("Bad Fats").** They increase the shelf life of food products but are not good for health.
  B. **Consume some omega-3 fatty acids every day ("Good Fats").** Only three grams a day may reduce risk of sudden cardiac death. As much as 50% to 80%, lower triglycerides and reduced inflammation may help prevent cancer. Include fish, e.g., salmon, mackerel and halibut – or take fish- or flaxseed-oil capsules from which contaminants have been removed.
  C. **Eat Less sugar and white flour**. They are low in fiber.

D. **Eat more fruits, vegetables, legumes and grains such as whole-wheat flour and brown rice**. They are rich in fiber, which slows absorption and fills up before taking in too many calories.

E. **Energy balance is important**. One loses weight when one burns calories.

F. **Exercise more and eat less**. Simple changes, taking the stairs, parking a little farther away and walking 30 minutes a day can make a difference. Small increases can lead to big improvements over time.

G. **Eat less red meat**. It's loaded with artery-clogging saturated fat and has been linked to an increased risk of cancer.

H. **Behavior modification**. Make lifestyle changes.

I. **Talk to suppliers.** Encourage food makers and restaurants to make it convenient and pleasurable to eat more healthfully.

J. **Choose quality over quantity**. Smaller portions of good foods are more satisfying than larger ports of fast foods.

REFERENCES

1. AACE/ACE Obesity Task Force. Position Statement on the Prevention, Diagnosis and Treatment of Obesity [online]. The American Association of Clinical Endocrinology, 1998 revision, www.aace.com/clinguideindex.htm
2. Adler, M, F Schaffner. Fatty liver hepatitis and cirrhosis in obese patients. Am J Med 1979; 67:811-816
3. Allen, JM, JI Koenig. Central and peripheral significance of neuropeptide Y and its related peptides. New York Academy of Sciences, 1990
4. Allison, DB, KR Fontaine, JE Manson, et al. Annual deaths attributable to obesity in the United States. JAMA 1999; 282:1530-1538
5. American Association of Clinical Endocrinologist and American College of Endocrinology. AACE/ACE Obesity Statement. Endo Prac 1997; 3:164-188
6. American College of Sports Medicine. **ACSM's Guidelines for Exercise Testing and Prescription**, 5th Edition. Baltimore, Williams and Wilkins, 1995
7. American Obesity Association. A pound of prevention for a healthier tomorrow. AOA Report. 1999, Vol 3, No 3
8. American Obesity Association. Minorities among the majority of obese. AOA Report. 1999, Vol 3, No 3
9. American Obesity Association. Is obesity a matter of genetics or behavior? AOA Report. 1999, Vol 3, No 3
10. American Obesity Association. New obesity cost study unveiled. AOA Report. 1999, Vol 3, No 3
11. American Obesity Association. Sizing the obesity public health message to fit obesity. AOA Report. 1999, Vol 3, No 3
12. American Obesity Association. Surgeon General ready to confront obesity Epidemic. AOA Report. 1999, Vol 3, No 3
13. American Obesity Association. What works in obesity treatment. AOA Report. 1999, Vol 3, No 3
14. Anderson, RE, CJ Crespo, SJ Barlett, et al. Relationship of physical activity and television watching with body weight and level of fatness among children: Results from the third national health and nutrition examination survey. JAMA 1998; 279(12):938-942
15. Angulo, P, J Keach, K Batts, K Lindo. Independent predictors or liver fibrosis in patients with nonalcoholic steatohepatitis. Hepatology 1999; 30:1356-1362

16. Bacon, B, M Farahvash, C Janney, B Neuschwander-Tetri. Nonalcoholic steatohepatitis: An expanded clinical entity. Gastroenterology 1994; 107:1103-1109
17. Balsiger, BM, FP Kennedy, HS Abu-Lebdeh, et al. Prospective evaluation of Rouz-en-Y gastric bypass as primary operation for medically complicated obesity. Mayo Clin Proc 2000; 75:673-680
18. Balsiger, BM, E Luque-de Leon, MG Sarr. Surgical treatment of obesity: Who is an appropriate candidate? Mayo Clinic Proc 1997; 72:551-558
19. Barsh, FS, IS Farooqi, S O'Rahilly. Genetics of body-weight regulation. Nature 2000; 404:644-651
20. Basaranoglu, M, O Aebay, A Sonsuz. A controlled trial of gemfibrozil in the treatment of patients with nonalcoholic steatohepatitis [Correespondence]. J Hepatol 1999; 31:384
21. Bellentani, S, G Saccoccio, F Masutti, et al. Prevalence of and risk factors for hepatic steatosis in Northern Italy. Ann Intern Med 2000; 132:112-117
22. Bennett, GA. Behavior therapy for obesity: A quantitative review of the effects of selected treatment characteristics on outcome. Behav Ther 1986; 17:554-562
23. Blackburn, GL. Functional foods in the prevention and treatment of disease: Significance of the dietary approaches to stop hypertension study. Am J Clin Nutr 1997; 66:1067-1071
24. Blumenkrantz, M. Obesity: The World's Oldest Metabolic Disorder."
25. Bonkovsky, H, Q Jawaid, K Tortorelli, et al. Non-alcoholic steatohepatitis and iron. Increased prevalence of mutations of the HFE gene in non-alcoholic steatohepatitis. J Hepatol 1999; 31:421-429
26. Boutelle, KN, DS Kirschenbaum. Further support for consistent self-monitoring as a vital component of successful weight control. Obes Res 1998; 6:219-224
27. Braillon, A, J Capron, M Nerve, et al. Liver in obesity. Gut 1985; 26:133-139
28. Brand-Miller, J, T Wolever, S Colagiuri, K Foster-Powell. The glucose Revolution: **The Authoritatie Guide to the Glycemic Index**. Marlowe & Company, New York, 1999.
29. Bray, GA, FL Greenway. Current and potential drugs for treatment of obesity. Endocrine Rev 1999; 20:805-875
30. Bray GA, J Leblanc, S Inoue, M Suzuki. **Diet and Obesity**. Japan Scientific Press, 1988

31. Bray, GA, LA Targaglia. Medicinal strategies in the treatment of obesity. Nature 2000; 404:672-677
32. Brolin, RE, RC Gorman, LM Milgrim, et al. Multivitamin prophylaxis in prevention of post-gastric bypass vitamin and mineral deficiencies. International Journal of Obesity 1991; 158:661-667
33. Brooks, D, RL Horner, LF Kozar, et al. Obstructive sleep apnea as a cause of systemic hypertension. Evidence from a canine model. J Clin Invest 1997; 99:106-109
34. Brownell, KN, DS Kirschenbaum. Exercise and obesity treatment: Psychological aspects. Int J Obes 1995; 19 (suppl 4):S122-S125
35. Brunt, E, C Janney, A Di Bisceglie, et al. Nonalcoholic steatohepatitis: A proposal for grading and staging the histological legions. Am J Gastroenterol 1999; 94:2467-2474
36. Caldwell, S, D Oelsner, J Iezzoni, et al. Cryptogenic cirrhosis: clinical characterization and risk factors for underlying disease. Hepatology 1999; 29:664-669
37. Centers for Disease Control. Prevalence of overweight and obesity among adults: United States, 1999. National Center for Health Statistics
38. Chandalia, M, A Garg, D Lutjohann, et al. Beneficial effects of high dietary fiber intake in patients with type 2 diabetes mellitus. NEJM 2000; 342(19):1392-1398
39. Chavin, K, S Yang, H Lin, et al. Obesity induces expression of uncoupling protein-2 in hepatocytes and promotes liver ATP depletion. J Biol Chem 1999; 274:5692-5700
40. Clark, CM. Diabetes. Primary Care 1999; 26(4):0095-4543
41. Colditz, GA. Economic costs of obesity and inactivity. Med Sci Sports Exercise 1999; 31:S669-S667
42. Cortez-Pinto, H, M Camilo, A Baptista, et al. Non-alcoholic fatty liver: Another feature of the metabolic syndrome? Clin Nutr 1999; 18:353-358
43. Cortez-Pinto, H, A Baptista, M Camilo, et al. Nonalcoholic steatohepatitis. Clinicopathological comparison with alcoholic hepatitis in ambulatory and hospitalized patients. Dig Dis Sci 1996; 41:172-179
44. Cortez-Pinto, H, J Chatham, V Chacko, et al. Alterations in liver ATP homeostasis in human nonalcoholic steatohepatitis – A pilot study. JAMA 1999; 282:1659-1664
45. Coulston, AM, CB Hollenbeck, MD Swislolock, et al. Effects of source of dietary carbohydrate on plasma glucose and insulin

responses to mixed meals in subjects with NIDDM. Diabetes Care 1987; 10:395-400

46. Day, C, O James. Steatohepatitis: A tale of two "hits"? [Editorial]. Gastroenterology 1998; 114:842-845
47. Diehl, A, Z Goodman, K Ishak. Alcohol-like liver disease in nonalcoholics. A clinical and histologic comparison with alcohol-induced liver injury. Gastroenterology 1988; 95:1056-1062
48. Diehl A. Nonalcoholic stearohepatitis. Sem Liv Dis 1999; 19:221-229
49. Drenick, E, F Simmons, J Murphy. Effect on hepatic morphology of treatment of obesity by fasting, reducing diets, and small-bowl bypass. N Engl J Med 1970; 282:829-834
50. Drerick, EJ, JJ Fisher. Sudden cardiac arrest in morbidly obese surgical patients unexplained after autopsy. Am J Surg 1988; 155: 720-726
51. Dyken, ME, VK Somers, T Yamada, et al. Investigating the relationship between stroke and obstructive sleep apnea. Stroke 1996; 27:401-407
52. Eriksson, S, K Eriksson, L Bondesson. Nonalcoholic seatohepatitis in obesity: A reversible condition. Acta Med Scand 1986; 220:83-88
53. Ewbank, PP, LL Darga, CP Lucas. Physical activity as a predictor of weight maintenance in previously obese subjects. Obesity Research 1995; 3(3):257-262
54. Federal Trade Commission. Consumer weight loss products and programs. What consumers stand to gain and lose. A public conference on the information consumers need to evaluate weight loss products and programs. Report of the presiding panel. Washington, DC: Federal Trade Commission, 1997
55. Ferguson, KA, T Ono, AA Lowe, et al. A short-term controlled trial of an adjustable oral appliance for the treatment of mild to moderate obstructive sleep apnea. Thorax 1997; 52:362-368
56. Flechtner-Mors M, H Ditschuneit, T Johnson, et al. Metabolic and weight-loss effects of long-term dietary intervention in obese patients: four-year results. Obes Res 2000; 8:399-402
57. Fontaine, KR, LJ Cheskin, and I Barofsky. Health related quality of life in obese persons seeking treatment. Journal of Family Practice 1996; 43(3):265-279
58. Foster-Powell, K, JC Brand Miller. International tables of Glycaemic Index. Am J Clin Nutr 1995; 62:871S-893S

59. Frank, A. Conflicts in the care of overweight patients: Inconsistent rules and insufficient money. Obesity Research 1997; 5(3):268-270
60. Friedman, JM, JL Halaas. Leptin and the regulation of body weight in mammals. Nature 1995; 395:763-770
61. Frost, G, J Wilding, J Beecham. Dietary advice based on glycaemic index improves dietary profile and metabolic control in Type 2 diabetic patients. Diabetic Med 1994; 11:397-401
62. Galuska, DA, JC Will, MK Serdula, ES Ford. Are health care professionals advising obese patients to lose weight? JAMA Association 282(16):1576-1578
63. Garcia-Monzon, C, E Martin-Perez, O Lo Iacono, et al. Characterization of pathogenic and prognostic factors of nonalcoholic steatohepatitis associated with obesity. J Hepatology 2000; 33:716-724
64. George, D, S Goldwurm, G MacDonald, et al. Increased hepatic iron concentration in nonalcoholic steatohepatitis is associated with increased fibrosis. Gastroenterology 1998; 114:311-318
65. Giacco, R, M Parillo, AA Rovellese, et al. Long-term dietary treatment with increased amounts of fiber-rich low glycemic index natural foods improves blood glucose control and reduces the number of hypoglycemic events in type 2 diabetic patients. Diabetes Care 2000; 23:1461-1466
66. Golan, M, A Weizman, M Fainaru. Impact of treatment for childhood obesity on parental risk factors for cardiovascular disease. Preventive Medicine 1999; 29(6):519-526
67. Gopalan, C, K Kamala. **Nutrition in Major Metabolic Diseases**. Delhi, India, Oxford University Press, 1997
68. Greenway, FL. Surgery for Obesity. Endocrinology and Metabolism Clinics of North America 1996; 25(4):1005-1027
69. Hall, JC, JM Watts, P O'Brien, et al. Gastric surgery for morbid obesity: the Adelaide Study. Annals of Surgery 1990; 211:419-437
70. Halsted, CH. Obesity: Effects on the liver and gastrointestinal system. Curr Opin Nutr Metab Care 199; 2:425-429
71. Havel, PJ, S Kassim-Karakas, W Mueller, et al. Relationship of plasma leptin to plasma insulin and adiposity in normal weight and overweight women: Effects of dietary fat content and sustained weight loss. J Clin Endocrinol Merab 1996; 81:4406-4413
72. Hensrud, D. **Mayo Clinic on Healthy Weight**. New York, NY, Kensington Publishing Corporation, 2000.
73. Hill, JO, FL Trowbridge. Childhood obesity: Future directions and research priorities. Pediatrics 1998; 101:570-574

74. Hill, JO. Dealing with obesity as a chronic disease. Obesity Research 1998; 6(1):34S-38S
75. Hsu, LKG, S Betancourt, SP Sullivan. Eating disturbances before and after vertical banded gastroplasty: A pilot study. International Journal of Eating Disorders. 1996; 19(1):23-24
76. Hung, J, EG Whitford, RW Parsons, et al. Association of sleep apnea with myocardial infarction in men. Lancet 1990; 336:261-264
77. Itoh, S, T Yougel, K Kawagoe. Comparison between nonalcoholic steatohepatitis and alcoholic hepatitis. Am J Gastroenterol 1987; 82: 650-654
78. Jorgensen, S, M Olesen, E Gudmand-Hoyer. A review of 20 years of jejunoileal bypass. Scand J Gastroenterol 1997; 32:334-339
79. Joseph, A, S Saverymuttu, S Al-Sam, et al. Comparison of liver histology with ultrasonography in assessing diffuse parenchymal liver disease. Clin Radiol 1991; 43:26-32
80. Kahn, HS, LM Tatham, C Rodriguez, et al. Stable behaviors associated with adults' 10-year change in body mass index and likelihood of gain at the waist. Am J Public Health 1997; 87:747-754
81. Kant, AK. Consumption of energy-dense, nutrient-poor foods by adult Americans: Nutritional and health implications. The third national health and nutrition examination survey, 1988-1994. Am J Clin Nutr 2000; 72(4):929-936
82. Kalarchian, MA, GT Wilson, RE Brolin, L Bradley. Binge eating in bariatric surgery patients. International Journal of Eating Disorders 1998; 23(1):89-92
83. Kaplan, LM. Genetics of obesity and body weight regulation. Cur Opin Endocrinol Diabetes 2000; 7:218-224
84. Kaplan, LM. Leptin, obesity and liver disease. Gastroenterology 1995; 115:997-1001
85. Keeffe, E, P Adesman, P Stenzel, R Palmer. Steatosis and cirrhosis in an obese diabetic. Resolution of fatty liver by fasting. Dig Dis Sci 1987; 32:441-445
86. Keim, NL, JS Stern PJ Havel. Relationship between circulating leptin concentrations and appetite during a prolonged, moderate energy deficit in women. Am J Clin Nutr 1998; 68:794-801
87. Khan, MA, J St Peter. Pharmacologic Therapy for Obesity. In: Gumbiner, B, Editor. **Obesity**. American College of Physicians, Philadelphia, PA, 2001, 221-254

88. Kohl, HK and KE Hobbs. Development of physical activity behaviors among children and adolescents. Pediatrics 1998; 101: 549-554
89. Kopelman, PG. Obesity as a medical problem. Nature 2000; 404:635-643
90. Kral, JG. Surgical treatment of obesity. In: Wadden, TA, TB VanItallie (Eds). **Treatment of the Seriously Obese Patient**. New York, Guilford Press, 1992, 496-506
91. Knol, JA. Management of the problem patient after bariatric surgery. Gastroenterology Clinics of North America 1994; 23(2):345-369
92. Kotz, CM, JE Briggs, JD Pomonis, et al. Neural site of leptin influence on neuropeptide Y signaling pathways altering feeding and uncoupling protein. Am J Physiol 1998; 275:R478-484
93. Kral, JG, LV Sjostrom, MBE Sullivan. Assessment of quality of life before and after surgery for severe obesity. American journal of Clinical Nutrition 1992; 55(2):611S-614S
94. Kribbs, NB, AI Pack, LR Kline, et al. Objective measurement of patterns of nasal CPAP use by patients with obstructive sleep apnea. Am Rev Respir Dis 1993; 147:887-889
95. Kuczmarski, RJ. Prevalence of overweight and weight gain in the United States. Am J Clinical Nutrition 1992; 55:495S-502S
96. Kuczmarski, RJ, KM Flegal, SM Campbell, et al. Increasing prevalence of overweight among US adults. JAMA 1994; 272:205-211
97. Kumanyika, SK. The impact of obesity on hypertension management in African Americans. Journal of Health Care for the Poor and Underserved 1997; 8(3):353
98. Kumanuika, SK. Special issues regarding obesity in minority populations. Annals of Internal Medicine 1993; 119(7pt2):650-654
99. Laurin, J, K Lindor, J Crippin, et al. Ursodeoxycholic acid or clofibrate in the treatment of non-alcohol-induced steatohepatitis: a pilot study. Hepatology 1996; 23:1464-1467
100. Lavine, J. Vitamin E treatment of nonalcoholic steatohepatitis in children: A pilot study. J Pediatr 2000; 136:734-738
101. Lee, R. Nonalcoholic steatohepatitis. A study of 45 patients. Hum Pathol 1989; 20:594-598
102. Matteoni, C, Z Younossi, T Gramlich, et al. Nonalcoholic fatty liver disease: A spectrum of clinical and pathological severity. Gastroenterology 1999; 116:1413-1419

103. Liu, S, J Manson, M Stampfer, et al. A Prospective Study of Whole-Grain Intake and Risk of Type 2 Diabetes Mellitus in US Women. Am J of Public Health 2000; 1409-1415
104. Luyckx, F, A Sheen, C Desaive, et al. Effects of gastroplasty on body weight and related biological abnormalities in morbid obesity. Diab Metab 1998; 24:355-361
105. McArthur, LH, JK Ross. Attitudes of registered dietitians toward personal overweight and overweight clients. Journal of the American Dietetics Association 1997; 97(1):63-66
106. McGarry, J, D Foster. Regulation of hepatic fatty acid oxidation and ketone body production. Annu Rev Biochem 1980; 49:395-420
107. McGinnis, JM and WH Foege. Actual causes of death in the United States. JAMA 1993; 270:2207-2212
108. Manson, JE, GA Colditz, MJ Stampfer, et al. A prospective study of obesity and risk of coronary heart disease in women. NEJM 1990; 322:882-889
109. Manson, JE, WC Willett, MJ Stampfer, et al. Body weight and mortality among women. NEJM 1995; 333:677-685
110. Marchesini, G, M Brizi, A Morselli-Labate, et al. Association of nonalcoholic fatty liver disease with insulin resistance. Am J Med 1999; 107:450-455
111. Meisler, JG, ST St Jeor. Summary and recommendations from the Amerian Health Foundations' expert panel of healthy weight. American Journal of Clinical Nutrition 1996; 63:474S-477S
112. Marceau, P, S Biron, F-S Hould. Liver pathology and the metabolic syndrome X in severe obesity. J Clin Endocrinol Metab 1999; 84:1513-1517
113. Mela, DJ. Determinants of food choice: Relationships with obesity and weight control. Obes Res 2001; Ssuppl 4:249S-255S
114. Methods for voluntary weight loss and control. NIH Technology Assess Statement Online 1992 Mar 30-April 1; (10)
115. Metz, JA, JS Stern, P Kris-Etherton, et al. A randomized trial of improved weight loss with a prepared meal plan in overweight and obese patients: Impact on cardiovascular risk reduction. Arch Intern Med 2000; (160):2150-2158
116. Meyer, JH. Nutritional outcomes of gastric operations. Gastroenterology Clinics of North America 1994; 23(2):227-230
117. Mezzanotte, WS, DJ Tangel and DP White. Waking and sleeping upper airway muscle activity in apnea patients versus normal controls. Am J Respir Crit Care Med 1996; 153:1880-1887

118. Mokdad, AH, MK Serdula, WH Dietz, et al. The spread of the obesity epidemic in the United States, 1991-1998. JAMA 1999; 282:1519-522
119. Mokdad, AH, MK Serdula, WH Dietz, et al. The continuing epidemic of obesity in the United States. JAMA 2000; 284:1650-1651
120. Moller, DE, AC Moses. Advances in the diagnosis and pathogenesis of diabetes mellitus and its complications. Comprehensive Medicine 1990; 16(7):41-48
121. Morin KH. Perinatal outcomes of obese women: A review of the literature. JOGNN 1998; 27(4):431-440
122. Nasrallah, S, C Wills, J Galambos. Hepatic morphology in obesity. Dig Dis Scil 1981; 26:325-327
123. Naslund E, L Beckman, L Granstrom, et al. Seven years results of vertical banding gastroplasty for morbid obesity. European Journal of Surgery 1997; 163:281-286
124. National Center for Health Statistics. Health United States 1998 with Socioeconomic Status and Health Chart Book. Hyattsville, MD: DHHS Publication Number (PHS) 1998; 98-1232
125. National Heart, Lung, and Blood Institute. Clinical Guidelines on the Identification, Evaluation, and Treatment of Obesity in Adults: The Evidence Report. NHLBI Obesity Education Initiative Expert Panel on the Identification, Evaluation, and Treatment of Obesity in Adults. Washington, DC. US Department of Health and Human Services, 1998
126. NIH Conference. Gastrointestinal surgery for severe obesity: Consensus development conference panel (review). Annals of Internal Medicine 1991; 115:956-961
127. National Institutes of Health, National Heart, Lung, and Blood Institute, North American Association for the Study of Obesity. The Practical Guide to the Identification, Evaluation, and Treatment of Overweight and Obesity in Adults. Bethesda, MD. October 2000. NIH Pub No. 00-4084
128. Office of Public Health and Service. Healthy People 2010 Objectives: Draft for Public Comment. Washington, DC. Department of Health and Human Services, Sept 1998
129. Pate RR, Health GW, M Dowda, SG Trost. Associations between physical activity and other health behaviors in a representative sample of US adolescents. Am J Public Health 1996; 86:1577-1581

130. Patton RW, JM Corry, LR Gettman, JS Graf. **Implementing Health/Fitness Programs**. Champaign, IL, Human Kinetics, 1986
131. Pennington, J. **Bowes and Church's Food Values of Portions Commonly Used**, 17th Edition. Philadelphia, Lippincott Ravens, 1998
132. Pi-Sunyer FX. Short-term medical benefits and adverse effects of weight loss. Annals of Internal Medicine 1993; 119:722-726
133. Pories, WJ, KG MacDonald, EJ Morgan, et al. Surgical treatment of obesity and its effect on diabetes: 10-year follow-up. American Journal of Clinical Nutrition 1992; 55:582S-585S
134. Position of the American Dietetic Association: Weight management. J Am Diet Assoc 1993; 97:71-74
135. Powell, E, W Cooksley, R Hanson, et al. The natural history of nonalcoholic steatohepatitis: A follow-up study of forty-two patients for up to 21 years. Hepatology 1990; 11:74-80
136. Powell NB, RW Riley, RJ Troell, et al. Radiofrequency volumetric tissue reduction of the palate in subjects with sleep-disordered breathing. Chest 1998; 113:1163-1174
137. Press Release. HHH News – DHHS, New Report Documents Improvement in Americans' Health. US Department of Health and Human Services, Washington, DC, June 10, 1999
138. Propst, A, T Propst, G Judmaier, W Vogel. Prognosis in nonalcoholic steatohepatitis (letter). Gastroenterology 1995; 108: 1607
139. Quesenberry, CP, B Caan, A Jacobson. Obesity, health services use, and health care costs among members of a health maintenance organization. Archives of Internal Medicine 1998; 158(9):466-472
140. Rabner, JG, S Dalton, RJ Greenstein. Obesity surgery: dietary and psychosocial expectations and reality. Mount Sinai Journal of Medicine 1993; 60(4):305-310
141. Rand, CSW, JM Kuldau, L Robbin. Surgery for obesity and marriage quality. JAMA 1982; 247:1419-1422
142. Rippe, JM. Overweight and health: Communications challenges and opportunities. American Journal of Clinical Nutrition 1996; 63(suppl):470S-473S
143. Rippe, J. The obesity epidemic: A mandate for a multidisciplinary approach. J Am Diet Assoc 1998; 98(suppl 2):5S-64S
144. Rosenbaum, M, R Leibel, J Hirsh. Obesity. NEJM 1997; 337: 396-407

145. Rothacker, DQ. Five-year self-management of weight using meal replacement: Comparison with matched controls in rural Wisconsin. Nutr 2000; 16:344-348
146. Sacks, FM, LP Svetkey, WM Vollmer, et al. Effects on blood pressure of reduced dietary sodium and the Dietary Approaches to Stop Hypertension (DASH) diet. DASH-Sodium Collaborative Research Group. NEJM 2001; 344(1):3-10
147. St Jeor, ST. New trends in weight management. Journal of the American Dietetic Association 1997; 97(10):1096-1098
148. St Peter, J, MA Khan. Obesity. In: DiPiro JT, Talbert RL, Yee GC, et al, (Eds). **Pharmacotherapy: A Pathophysiologic Appoach**. Fourth Edition. Stamford, CT, Appleton & Lange, 1999; 2334-2354
149. Sarlio-Lahteenkorva, S, A Stunkard, A Rissanen. Psychosocial factors and quality of life in obesity. International Journal of Obesity 1995; 19(6):S1-S5
150. Sheehan, JP. Update: NIDDM. Comprehensive Medicine 1990; 16(7):56-61
151. Shepard, RJ. Role of the physical activity in childhood obesity. Clin J Sports Med 2004; 14(3):161-180
152. Sher, AE, KB Schechtman, JF Piccirillo, et al. The efficacy of surgical modifications of the upper airway in adults with obstructive sleep apnea syndrome. Sleep 1996; 19:156-177
153. Shils, ME, JA Olson, M Shike, AC Ross, Editors. **Modern Nutrition in Health and Disease**. Ninth Edition. Philadelphia, Lippincott Williams & Wilkins 1999; 106-108
154. Siega-Riz, AM, LS Adair, CJ Hobel. Institute of Medicine maternal weight gain recommendations and pregnancy outcome in a predominantly Hispanic population. Obstetrics and Gynecology 1994; 84:565-573
155. Silverman, J, K O'Brien, S Long, et al. Liver pathology in morbidity obese patients with and without diabetes. Am J Gastroenterol 1990; 85:1349-1355
156. Simons-Morton, BG, WC Taylor, SA Snider, IW Huang. The physical activity of third-grade students during physical education classes. Am J Public Health 1993; 83:262-264
157. Simons-Morton, BG, WC Taylor, SA Snider, et al. Observed levels of elementary and middle school children's physical activity during physical education classes. Prev Med 1994; 23:437-441

158. Smith, PL, AR Gold, DA Meyers, et al. Weight loss in mildly to moderately obese patients with obstructive sleep apnea. Ann Intern Med 1985; 103:850-855
159. Solomon, CG, JE Manson. Obesity and mortality: A review of the epidemiologic data. Am J Clin Nutr 1997; 66:1044S-1050S
160. Tajiri, K, H Takenawa, K Yamaoka, et al. Nonalcoholic steatohepatitis masquerading as autoimmune hepatitis. J Clin Gastroenterol 1997; 25:538-540
161. Tankurt, E, S Biberoglu, E Ellidokuz, et al. Hyperinsulinemia and insulin resistance in non-alcoholic steatohepatitis. J Hepatol 1999; 31:963
162. Teran-Santos, J, A Jimenez-Gomez, J Cordero-Guevara, et al. The association between sleep apnea and the risk of traffic accidents. NEJM 1999; 340:847-851
163. Tierney, LM, SJ McPhee, MA Papdakis, Editors. **Current Medical Diagnosis and Treatment**. Stamford, CT, Appleton and Lange, 1998; 161-1164
164. Tomeo, CA, AE Field CS Berkey. Weight concerns, weight control behaviors, and smoking cessation. Pediatrics 1999; 104(4): 918-924
165. Troiano, RP, KM Flegal. Overweight children and adolescents: Description, epidemiology, and demographics. Pediatrics 1998; 101(3):497-504
166. Tucker, LA, GM Friedman. Obesity and absenteeism: An epidemiologic study of 10,825 employed adults. American Journal of Health Promotion 1998; 12(3):202-207
167. US Department of Health and Human Services. 1992 National Survey of Worksite Health Promotion Activities Summary Report. Washington, DC, US Government Printing Office, 1993
168. Van Itallie, TB. Health implications of overweight and obesity in the United States. Annals of Internal Medicine. 1985; 103(6(Part 2)):983-988
169. Van Ness, M, A Diehl. Is liver biopsy useful in the evaluation of patients with chronically elevated liver enzymes? Ann Intern Med 1989; 111:473-478
170. Van Steenbergen, W, S Lanchkmans. Liver disturbances in obesity and diabetes mellitus. Internation J Obesity 10995; 19:S27-S36
171. Ratziu, V, P Giral, F Charlotte, et al. Liver fibrosis in overweight patients. Gastroenterology 2000; 118:1117-1123
172. Vuksan, V, D Jenkins, P Spadafora et al. Konjac-Mannan (Glucomannan) inproves glycemic and other associated risk factors

for coronary heart disease in type 2 diabetes. Diabetes Care 2000; 22(6):913-918
173. Vuksan, V, J Sievenpiper, R Owen, et al. Beneficial effects of viscous dietary fiber from Konjac-Mannan in Subjects with the insulin resistance syndrome. Diabetes Care 2000; 23(1):9-13
174. Wadden, TA, RI Berkowitz, RA m Vogt, et al. Lifestyle modification in the pharmacologic treatment of obesity: A pilot investigation of a potential primary care approach. Obes Res 1997; 5:218-226
175. Waller, DK, JL Mills, JL Simpson, et al. Are obese women at higher risk for producing malformed offspring? American Journal of Obstetrics and Gynecology 1994; 170:541-548
176. Weinsier, RL. Etiology of the increasing prevalence of obesity among US adults. Obes Res 1997; 5(suppl 1):95S
177. Weltman, M, G Farrell, P Hall, et al. Hepatic cytochrome P450 2E1 is increased in patients with nonalcoholic steatohepatitis. Hepatology 1998; 27:128-133
178. Wheatley, JR, WS Mezzanotte, DJ Tangel, DP White. Influence of sleep on genioglossal muscle activation by negative pressure in normal men. Am Rev Resp Dis 1993; 148:597-605
179. Willett, WC, WH Dietz, GA Colditz. Guidelines for healthy weight. NEJM 1999; 341:427-434
180. Williams, MV, DW Bake, RM Parker, JR Nurss. Relationship of functional healthiteracy to patients' knowledge of their chronic disease: A study of patients with hypertension and diabetes. Archives of Internal Medicine 1998; 158:166-172
181. Williamson, DF, J Madans, RF Anda, et al. Smoking cessation and severity of weight gain in a national cohort. NEJM 1991; 324(11): 739-745
182. Wilson, GT. Acceptance and change in the treatment of eating disorders and obesity. Behavior Therapy 1996; 27:417-439
183. Wolever, T. The Glycemic index: Flogging a dead horse? Diabetes Care 1997; 20(3)452-456
184. Wolf, AM, GA Colditz. Current estimates of the economic cost of obesity in the United States. Obesity Research 1998; 6(2):97-106
185. World Health Organization. Obesity: Preventing and Managing the Global Epidemic. Report of the WHO Consultation on Obesity. Geneva, World Health Organization, 1997
186. Wright J, R Johns, I Watt, et al. Health effects of obstructive sleep apnea and the effectiveness of continuous positive airway pressure:

A systematic review of the research evidence. BMJ 1997; 314:851-860

187. Yang, S, H Lin, M Lane, et al. Obesity increases sensitivity to endotoxin liver injury: Implications for the pathogenesis of steatohepatitis. Proc Natl Acad Sci USA 1997; 94:2557-2562
188. Young, T, P Peppard, M Palta, et al. Population-based study of sleep disordered breathing as a risk factor for hypertension. Arch Intern Med 1997; 157:1746-1752

Appendices

APPENDIX I

THE WEIGHT-REDUCTION READINESS TEST

For each question, circle the answer that best describes your attitude, then write the number of your answer on the line before each question number.

Section 1: Goals and Attitudes

(1) Never; (2) Rarely; (3) Occasionally; (4) Frequently; (5) Always

___ 1. Compared to previous attempts, how motivated are you to lose weight at this time?

a. Extremely motivated
b. Quite motivated
c. Somewhat motivated
d. Slightly motivated
e. Not at all motivated

___ 2. How certain are you that you will stay committed to a weight-loss program for the time it will take to reach your goal?

1. Extremely certain
2. Quite certain
3. Somewhat certain
4. Slight certain
5. Not at all certain

___ 3. Consider all outside factors at this time in your life. To what extent can you tolerate the effort required to stick to a program?

1. Can tolerate easily
2. Can tolerate well
3. Uncertain
4. Can tolerate
5. Cannot tolerate

___ 4. Figuring a weight loss of two pounds per week, how realistic is your expectation?

1. Very realistic
2. Somewhat realistic

3. Moderately realistic
4. Somewhat unrealistic
5. Very unrealistic

___ 5. While losing weight, do you dream about eating a lot of your favorite foods?
1. Never
2. Rarely
3. Occasionally
4. Frequently
5. Always

______ **Section 1** _____ **TOTAL Score**

If you scored:

1 to 8:	Very motivated
9 to 16:	Moderate motivated
17 to 25:	It may not be a good time to start weight loss program

Section 2: Hunger and External Eating Cues

___ 1. Do you want to eat even if you are not hungry?
1. Never
2. Rarely
3. Occasionally
4. Frequently
5. Always

___ 2. How often do you eat because of physical hunger?
1. Always
2. Frequently
3. Occasionally
4. Rarely
5. Never

___ 3. Do you have trouble controlling your eating when your favorite foods are around the house?
1. Never
2. Rarely

3. Occasionally
4. Frequently
5. Always

______ **Section 2** _____ **TOTAL Score**

If you scored:

1 to 8: You might occasionally eat more than you would like, but it does not appear to be a result of high responsiveness to external cues.

7 to 9: You may have a moderate tendency to eat just because food is available.

10 to 15: Some or most of your eating may be in response to thinking about food or exposing yourself to temptations to eat.

Section 3: Control over Eating

If the following situations occurred while you were on a weight-loss program, would you be likely to eat more or less immediately afterward and for the rest of the day?

___ 1. Although you planned on skipping lunch, a friend talks you into going out for a meal.
1. Would eat much less
2. Would eat somewhat less
3. Would make no difference
4. Would eat somewhat more
5. Would eat much more

___ 2. You "break" your diet by eating "forbidden" food.
1. Would eat much less
2. Would eat somewhat less
3. Would make no difference
4. Would eat somewhat more
5. Would eat much more

___ 3. You have been following your diet faithfully and decide to test yourself by eating something you consider a treat.
1. Would eat much less
2. Would eat somewhat less
3. Would make no difference
4. Would eat somewhat more
5. Would eat much more

______ **Section 3** _____ **TOTAL Score**

If you scored:

3 to 7: You recover rapidly from mistakes.

8 to 11: You do not seem to let unplanned eating disrupt your program.

12 to 15: You may be prone to overeat after an event breaks your control or throws you off the track.

Section 4: Binge Eating and Purging

___ 1. Aside from holiday feasts, have you ever eaten a large amount of food rapidly and felt afterward that this eating incident was excessive and out of control?
2 Yes
0 No

___ 2. If you answered yes to question 1 above, how often have you engaged in this behavior during the last year?
1. Less tan once a month
2. About once a month
3. A few times a month
4. About once a week
5. About three times a week
6. Daily

___ 3. Have you ever purged (used laxatives, diuretics or induced vomiting) to control your weight?
5 Yes
0 No

___ 4. If you answered yes to question 3 above, how often have you engaged in this behavior during the last year?
   1. Less than once a month
   2. About once a month
   3. A few times a month
   4. About once a week
   5. About three times a week
   6. Daily

______ **Section 3** _____ **TOTAL Score**

If you scored:

0 to 1: It appears that binge eating and purging is not a problem for you.

2 to 11: Pay attention to these eating patterns.

12 to 19: You show signs of having a potentially serious eating problem.

Section 5: Exercise Patterns

___ 1. How often do you exercise?
   1. Never
   2. Rarely
   3. Occasionally
   4. Frequently
   5. Always

___ 2. How confident are you that you can exercise regularly?
   1. Not at all confident
   2. Slightly confident
   3. Somewhat confident
   4. Quite confident
   5. Extremely confident

___ 3. When you think about exercise, do you develop a positive or negative picture in your mind?
   1. Completely negative

2. Somewhat negative
3. Neutral
4. Somewhat positive
5. Completely positive

___ 4. How certain are you that you can work regular exercise into your daily schedule?
1. Not at all certain
2. Slightly certain
3. Somewhat certain
4. Quite certain
5. Extremely certain

______ **Section 6** _____ **TOTAL Score**

If you scored:

4 to 10: You are probably not exercising as regularly as you should.

11 to 16: You need to feel more positive about exercise so you can do it more often.

APPENDIX II

NUTRITIONAL ASSESSMENT

Name________________________________ Gender: ❑Male ❑Female

Date of Birth ___/___/___ Height _____ Weight _____ Goal _____

Body Mass Index (BMI)__________Waist Circumference __________

Hip Circumference ____________ Waist/Hip Ratio (WHR) __________

Medical Problems ____

Medication (prescribed) _______________________________________

Medications (over-the-counter) __________________________________

____

Herbs ____

Vitamins ____

Lab Values: Total Cholesterol _____ HDL-C _____ LDL-C ______

Triglycerides ______ Glucose ______

Other Lab values: ____

Weight Reduction Readiness Test (answers to some questions)

1. Motivation
2. Stress
3. Control Overeating
4. Binge Eating
5. Exercise Patterns

Previous Weight Reduction Diet _________________________________

Comments: ____

Weight Management Prescription

Diet Therapy ____

Exercise Recommendations ______________________________

Behavior Modifications __________________________________

Other Recommendations (e.g., meal replacement and/or drug therapy)

____

APPENDIX III

FOOD DIARY

				Today's Date: ____________
Description	**Time**	**Feelings**	**Activity**	**Calories**
Breakfast				
Total calories from this meal				
Lunch				
Total calories from this meal				
Dinner				
Total calories from this meal				
Snacks				
Total calories from snacks				
Total calories for the day				

APPENDIX IV

BEHAVIOR MODIFICATION STRATEGIES

1. Keep an eating diary
2. Maximize awareness of eating
3. Examine patterns in your eating
4. Prevent automatic eating
5. Identify triggers for eating
6. Do nothing else while eating (e.g., watching TV)
7. Follow an eating schedule
8. Eat in one place
9. Do not clean your plate
10. Put your fork down between bites
11. Pause during the meal
12. Shop on a full stomach
13. Shop from a list
14. Buy foods that require preparation
15. Keep problem food out of sight
16. Keep healthy foods visible
17. Remove serving dishes from table
18. Leave the table after eating
19. Serve and eat one portion at a time
20. Avoid being a food dispenser
21. Use alternatives to eating
22. Use strategies for eating away from home
23. Prepare in advance for special events
24. Plan in advance for high-risk situations
25. Identify your behavior chains
26. Interrupt your behavior chains
27. Set realistic goals

APPENDIX V

WAYS TO SIZE UP SERVINGS

Measure food portions so you know exactly how much food you're eating. When a food scale or measuring cups aren't handy, you can still estimate your portion. Remember:

3 ounces of meat is about the size and thickness of a deck of playing cards or an audiotape cassette.	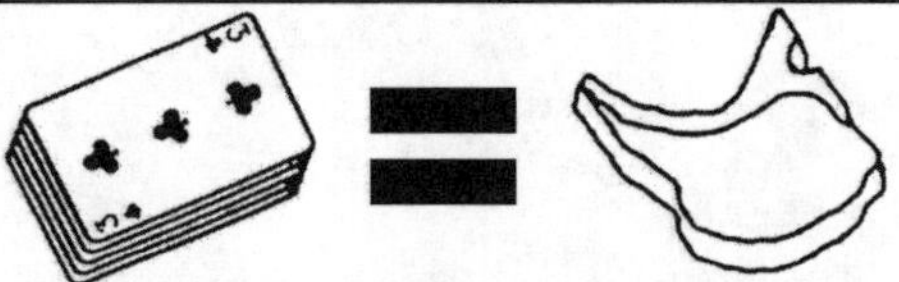
a medium apple or peach is about the size of a tennis ball.	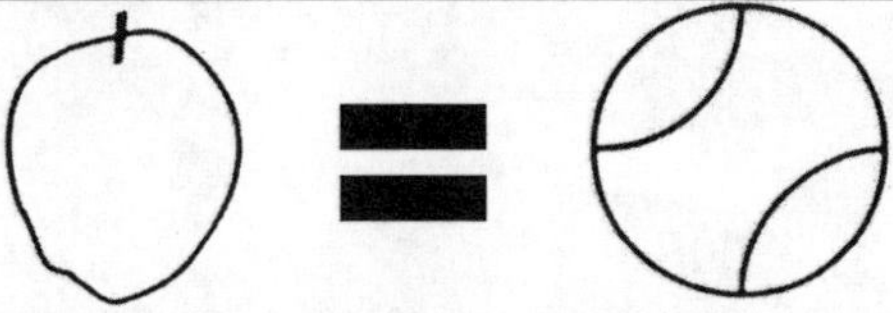
one oz of cheese is about the size of 4 stacked dice.	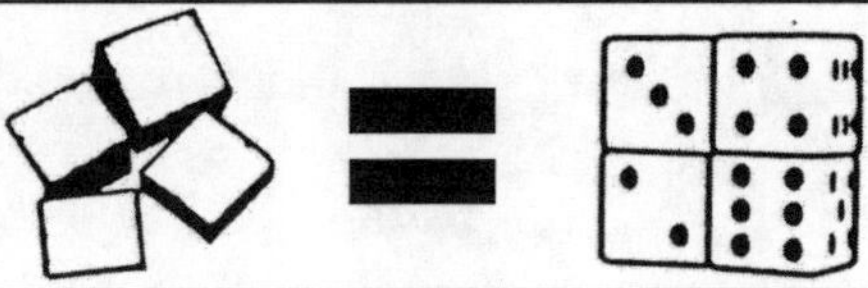
½ cup of ice cream is about the size of a racquetball or tennis ball.	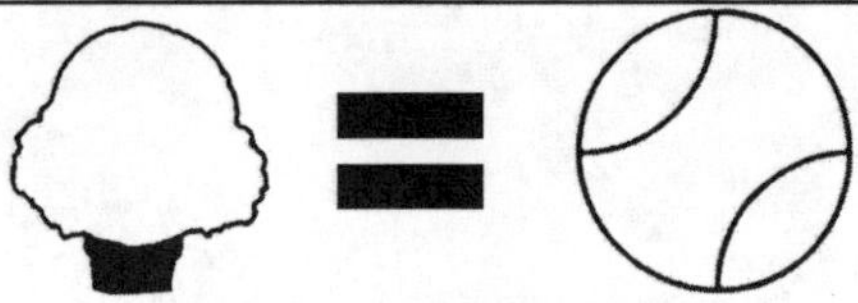
one cup of mashed potatoes or broccoli is about the size of your fist.	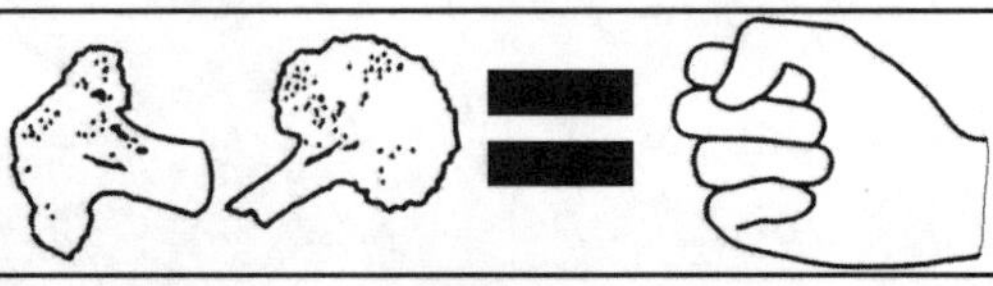
one teaspoon of butter or peanut butter is about the size of the tip of your thumb.	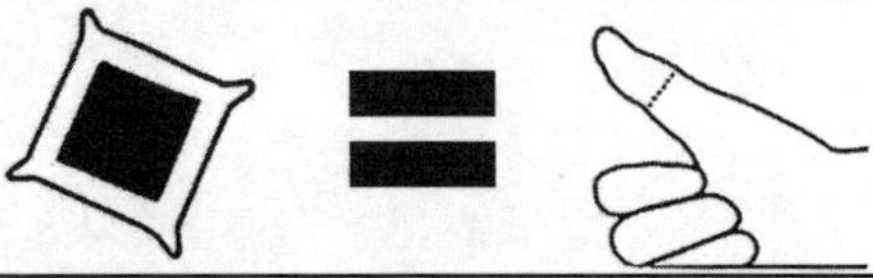
one ounce of nuts or small candies equals one handful.	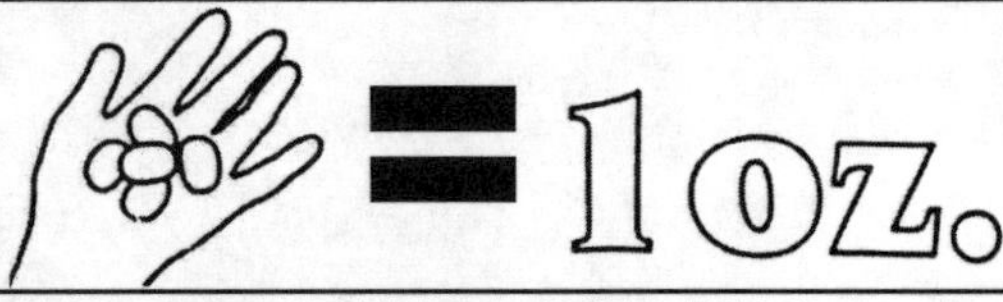

Source: *National Dairy Council, Rosemont, Illinois 60018-5616*

APPENDIX VI

GENERAL GUIDELINES FOR EXERCISING

CHOOSING THE BEST ACTIVITY

There are many activities to choose from. There are four factors to consider in making your decision.

1. **Select Something You Can Do.** Consider your current physical condition when choosing an activity. Basketball is strenuous and is not advisable if you are not in tip-top condition. Pick something where you can move at your own pace. Walking, cycling, and swimming are good examples.

2. **Select Something You Would Like To Do.** Hiking may be something that always caught your fancy, so go ahead and try. If you are turned off by swimming, don't do it just because you think you should. It helps to like the activity you choose.

3. **Select a Solo or Social Activity.** We covered this earlier in our discussion of walking. In your choice of an activity, consider whether you would like to exercise along (jogging, swimming, cycling) or with other people (tennis, golf, aerobics class). If you are a special person, having others around can be an incentive to participate.

4. **Do Not Be Embarrassed**. This is easier said than done. Many dieters avoid exercise completely or avoid it when they can be seen by others.

APPENDIX VII

EXERCISE AND CALORIES CHART

The chart below shows the approximate calories burned by a 150 pound woman. If you weigh less, you will burn fewer calories; if you weight more, you will burn more.

Approximate calories burned, per hour by a 150 pound women

Type of Exercise	Calories/hour
Sleeping	55
Eating	85
Sewing	85
Knitting	85
Sitting	85
Standing	100
Driving	110
Office work	140
Housework, moderate	160+
Golf, with trolley	180
Golf, without trolley	240
Gardening, planting	250
Dancing, ballroom	260
Walking, 3mph	280
Table tennis	290
Garden, hoeing, etc.	350
Tennis	350+
Water aerobics	400
Skating/blading	420+
Dancing, aerobic	420+
Aerobic	450+
Jogging, 5mph	500
Gardening, digging	500
Swimming, active	500+
Cross country ski machine	500+
Hiking	500+
Step aerobics	550+

Rowing	550+
Power walking	600+
Cycling, studio	650
Squash	650+
Skipping with rope	700+
Running	700+

APPENDIX VIII

FOOD EXCHANGE LIST

Within each group, these foods can be exchanged for each other. You can use this list to give yourself more choices.

Vegetables contain 25 calories and 5 grams of carbohydrate. One serving equals:

- ½ cup — Cook vegetables (carrots, broccoli, zucchini, cabbage, etc.)
- 1 cup — Raw vegetables of salad greens
- ½ cup — Vegetable juice

If you're hungry, eat more fresh or steamed vegetables.

Fat Free and Very Low Fat Milk contains 90 calories and 12 grams of carbohydrate per serving. One serving equals:

- 8 oz — Milk, fat free or 1% fat
- 3/4 cup — Yogurt, plain nonfat or lowfat
- 1 cup — Yogurt, artificially sweetened

Very Lean Protein choices have 35 calories and 1 gram of fat per serving. One serving equals:

- 1 oz — Turkey breast or chicken breast, skin removed
- 1 oz — Fish fillet (flounder, sole, scrod, cod, haddock, halibut)
- 1 oz — Canned tuna in water
- 1 oz — Shellfish (clams, lobster, scallop, shrimp)
- 3/4 cup — Cottage cheese, nonfat or lowfat
- 2 each — Egg whites
- 1/4 cup — Egg substitute
- 1 oz — Fat free cheese
- ½ cup — Beans - cooked (black beans, kidney, chickpeas, or lentils): count as 1 starch/bread and 1 very lean protein

Fruits contain 15 grams of carbohydrates and 60 calories. One serving equals:

- 1 small apple, banana, orange, nectarine
- 1 medium fresh peach
- 1 Kiwi
- ½ Grapefruit
- ½ Mango
- 1 cup Fresh berries (strawberries, raspberries, or blueberries)
- 1 cup Fresh melon cubes
- 1/4 Honeydew melon
- 4 oz Unsweetened juice
- 4 tsp Jelly or jam

Lean Protein choices have 55 calories and 2 to 3 grams of fat per serving. One serving equals:

- 1 oz Chicken - dark meat, skin removed
- 1 oz Turkey - dark meat, skin removed
- 1 oz Salmon, swordfish, herring, catfish, trout
- 1 oz Lean beef (flank steak, London broil, tenderloin, roast beef)*
- 1 oz Veal, roast, or lean chop*
- 1 oz Lamb, roast, or lean chop*
- 1 oz Pork, tenderloin, or fresh ham*
- 1 oz Lowfat cheese (3 grams or less of fat per ounce)
- 1 oz 4.5% cottage cheese
- 2 medium Sardines

*Limit to 1 to 2 times per week.

Medium Fat Proteins have 75 calories and 5 grams of fat per serving. One serving equals:

- 1 oz Beef (any prime cut), corned beef, ground beef**
- 1 oz Pork Chop
- 1 each Whole egg (medium) **
- 1 oz Mozzarella cheese
- 1/4 cup Ricotta cheese
- 4 oz Tofu (note that this is a heart-healthy choice)

**Choose these very infrequently.

Starches contain 15 grams of carbohydrate and 80 calories per serving. One serving equals:

- 1 slice Bread (white, pumpernickel, whole wheat, rye
- 2 slices Reduced calorie or "lite" bread
- 1/4 (1 oz) Bagel (varies)
- ½ English muffin
- ½ Hamburger bun
- 3/4 cup Cold cereal
- 1/3 cup Rice, brown or white - cooked
- 1/3 cup Barley or couscous - cooked
- 1/3 cup Legumes (dried beans, peas, or lentils) - cooked
- ½ cup Pasta-cooked
- ½ cup Bulgur - cooked
- ½ cup Corn, sweet potato, or green peas
- 3 oz Baked sweet or white potato
- 3/4 oz Pretzels
- 3 cups Popcorn, hot-air popped or microwave (80-percent light)

Fats contain 45 calories and 5 grams of fat per serving. One serving equals:

- 1 tsp Oil (vegetable, corn, canola, olive, etc.)
- 1 tsp Butter
- 1 tsp Stick Margarine
- 1 tsp Mayonnaise
- 1 T Reduced fat margarine or mayonnaise
- 1 T Salad dressing
- 1 T Cream cheese
- 2 T Lite cream cheese
- 1/8 Avocado
- 8 large Black olives
- 10 large Stuffed green olives
- 1 slice Bacon

Source: *NIH Publication, Number 00-4084, October 2000*

APPENDIX IX

SUBSTITUTION OF HIGH CALORIE FOODS WITH LOW CALORIE FOODS

These low calorie alternatives provide new ideas for old favorites. When making a food choice, remember to consider vitamins and minerals. Some foods provide most of their calories from sugar and fat but give you few, if any, vitamins and mineral.

This guide is not meant to be an exhaustive list. We stress reading labels to find out just how many calories are in the specific products you decide to buy.

Instead of	Replace with . . . . . .
• Evaporated whole milk	• Evaporated fat free (skim) or reduced fat (2%) milk
• Whole milk	• Lowfat (1%), reduced fat (2%), or fat free (skim) milk
• Ice cream	• Sorbet, sherbet, lowfat or fat free frozen yogurt, or ice milk (check label for calorie content)
• Whipping cream	• Imitation whipped cream (made with fat free [skim] milk) or lowfat vanilla yogurt
• Sour cream, Cream cheese	• Plain lowfat yogurt, Neufchatel or "light" cream cheese or fat free cream cheese
• Cheese (cheddar, Swiss, jack)	• Reduced calorie cheese, low calorie processed cheeses, etc., Fat free cheese
• American cheese	• Fat free American cheese or other types of fat free cheeses

• Regular (4%) cottage cheese	• Lowfat (1%) or reduced fat (2%) cottage cheese
• Whole milk mozzarella cheese	• Part skim milk, low-moisture mozzarella cheese
• Whole milk ricotta cheese	• Part skim milk ricotta cheese
• Coffee cream (half and half) or nondairy creamer (liquid, powder)	• Lowfat (1%) or reduced fat (2%) milk or nonfat dry milk powder
• Ramen noodles	• Rice or noodles (spaghetti, macaroni, etc.)
• Pasta with white sauce (alfredo)	• Pasta with red sauce (marinara)
• Pasta with cheese sauce	• Pasta with vegetables (primavera) • Bran flakes, crispy rice, etc. • Cooked grits or oatmeal • Whole grains (e.g., couscous, barley, bulgur, etc.)
• Granola	• Reduced fat granola
• Cold cuts, lunch meats (bologna, salami, liverwurst, etc.)	• Lowfat cold cuts (95% to 97% fat free lunch meats, lowfat pressed meats)
• Hot dogs (regular)	• Lower fat hot dogs
• Bacon or sausage	• Canadian bacon or lean ham
• Regular ground beef	• Extra lean ground beef such as ground round or ground turkey (read labels)
• Chicken or turkey with skin, duck, or goose	• Chicken or turkey without skin (white meat)
• Oil-packed tuna	• Water-packed tuna (rinse to reduce sodium content)
• Beef (chuck, rib, brisket)	• Beef (round, loin) (trimmed of external fat) (choose select grades)

• Pork (spareribs, untrimmed loin)	• Pork tenderloin or trimmed, lean smoked ham
• Frozen breaded fish or fried fish (homemade or commercial)	• Fish or shellfish, unbreaded (fresh, frozen, canned in water
• Whole eggs	• Egg whites or egg substitutes
• Frozen TV dinners (containing more than 13 grams of fat per serving)	• Frozen TV dinners (containing less than 13 grams of fat per serving and lower in sodium)
• Chorizo sausage	• Turkey sausage, drained well (read label) • Vegetarian sausage (made with tofu)
• Croissants, brioches, etc.	• Hard french rolls or soft "brown 'n serve" rolls
• Donuts, sweet rolls, muffins, scones, or pastries	• English muffins, bagels, reduced fat or fat free muffins or scones
• Party crackers	• Lowfat crackers (choose lower in sodium)
• Cake (pound, chocolate, yellow)	• Saltine or soda crackers (choose lower in sodium)
• Cookies	• Cake (angel food, white, gingerbread) • Reduced fat or fat free cookies (graham crackers, ginger snaps, fig bars) (compare calorie level)
• Nuts	• Popcorn (air-popped or light microwave), fruits, vegetables
• Ice cream, e.g., cones or bars	• Frozen yogurt/fruit, or chocolate pudding bars
• Custards or puddings (made with whole milk)	• Puddings (made with skim milk)

• Regular margarine or butter	• Light-spread margarines, diet • margarine, or whipped butter, tub or squeeze bottle
• Regular mayonnaise	• Light or diet mayonnaise or mustard
• Regular salad dressings	• Reduced calorie or fat free salad dressings, lemon juice, or plain, herb-flavored, or wine vinegar
• Butter or margarine on toast or bread	• Jelly, jam, or honey on bread or toast
• Oils, shortening, or lard	• Nonstick cooking spray for stir-frying or sautéing as a substitute for oil or butter, use applesauce or prune puree in baked goods
• Canned cream soups	• Canned broth-based soups
• Canned beans and franks	• Canned baked beans in tomato sauce
• Gravy (homemade with fat and/ or milk)	• Gravy mixes made with water or homemade with the fat skimmed off and fat free milk included
• Fudge sauce	• Chocolate syrup
• Avocado on sandwiches	• Cucumber slices or lettuce leaves
• Guacamole dip or refried beans with lard	• Salsa

Source: *NIH Publication #00-4084, October 2000*

APPENDIX X

SAMPLE REDUCED CALORIE MENUS

Traditional American Cuisine - 1,200 Calories You can use the exchange list in Appendix VIII to give yourself more choices.				
	Calories	**Fat (grams)**	**% Fat**	**Exchange for:**
Breakfast				
- Whole wheat bread, 1 medium slice	70	1.2	15	**(One bread/ starch)**
- Jelly, regular, 2 tsp	30	0	0	**(½ fruit)**
- Cereal, shredded wheat, ½ cup	104	1	4	**(one bread/**
- Milk, 1%, 1 cup	102	3	23	**starch)**
- Orange juice, 3/4 cup	78	0	0	**(one milk)**
- Coffee, regular, 1 cup	5	0	0	**(1 ½ fruit)**
Breakfast Total	**389**	**5.2**	**10**	**(Free)**
Lunch				
- Roast beef sandwich:				
Whole wheat bread, 2 medium slices	139	2.4	15	**(2 bread/ starch) (2 lean protein)**
Lean roast beef, unseasoned, 2 oz	60	105	23	**(1 vegetable)**
Lettuce, 1 leaf	1	0	0	**(1/3 fat)**
Tomato, 3 medium slices	10	0	0	**(1 fruit)**
Mayonnaise, low calorie, 1 tsp	15	1.7	96	**(free)**
- Apple, 1 medium	80	0	0	
- Water, 1 cup	0	0	0	
Lunch Total	**305**	**5.6**	**16**	
Dinner				
- Salmon, 2 ounces edible	103	5	44	**(2 lean protein)**
- Vegetable oil, 1 ½ tsp	60	7	100	**(1 ½ fat)**
- Baked potato, 3/4 medium	100	0	0	**(bread/starch)**
- Margarine, 1 tsp	34	4	100	**(1 fat)**
- Green beans, seasoned, with margarine, ½ cup	52	2	4	**(1 vegetable) (½ fat)**
- Carrots, sesoned	35	0	0	**(1 vegetable)**
- White dinner roll, 1 small	70	2	28	**(1 bread/ starch)**
- Iced tea, unsweetened, 1 cup	0	0	0	**(free)**
- Water, 2 cups	0	0	0	**(free)**
Dinner Total	**454**	**20**	**39**	

Snack - Popcorn, 2 ½ cups - Margarine, 3/4 tsp	 69 30	 0 3	 0 100	 **(1 bread/ starch)** **(3/4 fat)**
TOTAL	**1,247**	**34-36**	**24-26**	

Calories..1,247
Total carbohydrate, % kcals...............58
Total fat, % kcals...............................26
*Sodium, mg.................................1,043
Saturated fat, % Kcals........................7
Cholesterol, mg.................................96
Protein, % kcal 19

Note: Calories have been rounded.

1,200: 100% RDA met for all nutrients except vitamin E 80%, vitamin B_2, 96%, vitamin B_6 94%, calcium 68%, iron 63%, zinc 73%.

*No salt added in recipe preparation or as seasoning. Consume at least 32 ounces of water.

Asian American Cuisine - Reduced Calorie		
Breakfast	**1,600 Calories**	**1,200 Calories**
- Banana	1 small	1 small
- Whole wheat bread	2 slices	1 slice
- Margarine	1 tsp	1 tsp
- Orange juice	3/4 cup	3/4 cup
- Milk 1%, lowfat	3/4 cup	3/4 cup
Lunch		
- Beef noodle soup, canned, low sodium	1/2 cup	½ cup
- Chinese noodle and beef salad:		
Roast beef	3 oz	2 oz
Peanut oil	1 ½ tsp	1 tsp
Soy sauce, low sodium	1 tsp	1 tsp
Carrots	½ cup	½ cup
Zucchini	½ cup	½ cup
Onion	1/4 cup	1/4 cup
Chinese noodles, soft type	1/4 cup	1/4 cup
- Apple	1 medium	1 medium
- Tea, unsweetened	1 cup	1 cup
Dinner		
- Pork stir-fry with vegetables		
Pork cutlet	2 oz	2 oz
Peanut oil	1 tsp	1 tsp
Soy sauce, low sodium	1 tsp	1 tsp
Broccoli	½ cup	½ cup
Carrots	1 cup	½ cup

Mushrooms	1/4 cup	½ cup
- Steamed white rice	1 cup	½ cup
- Tea, unsweetened	1 cup	1 cup
Snack		
- Almond cookies	2 cookies	-
- Milk 1%, lowfat	3/4 cup	3/4 cup

Calories....................................1,609
Total carbohydrate, % kcals...........56
Total fat, % kcals...........................27
*Sodium, mg.............................1,296
Saturated fat, % kcals........8
Cholesterol, mg.............148
Protein, % kcals..............20

Calories...................................1,220
Total Carbohydrates, % kcals........55
Total fat, % kcals...........................27
*Sodium, mg...........................1,043
Saturated fat, % kcals......................8
Cholesterol, mg..........................117
Protein, % kcals......................... 21

1,600:100% RDA met for all nutrients except zinc 95%, iron 87%, and calcium 93%
1,200:100% RDA met for all nutrients except vitamin E 75%, calcium 84%, magnesium 98%, iron 66%, and zinc 77%.
*No salt added in recipe preparation or as seasoning. Consume at least 32 ounces of water.

Southern Cuisine - Reduced Calorie		
Breakfast	**1,600 Calories**	**1,200 Calories**
- Oatmeal, prepared with 1% milk, lowfat	½ cup	½ cup
- Milk, 1%, lowfat	½ cup	½ cup
- English muffin	1 medium	-
- Cream cheese, light, 18% fat	1 T	-
- Orange juice	3/4 cup	½ cup
- Coffee	1 cup	1 cup
- Milk, 1%, lowfat	1 oz	1 oz
Lunch		
-Baked chicken, without skin	1/2 cup	½ cup
-Vegetable oil		
- Salad:		
Lettuce	3 oz	2 oz
Tomato	1 ½ tsp	1 tsp
Cucumber	1 tsp	1 tsp
- Oil and vinegar dressing	½ cup	½ cup
- White rice	½ cup	½ cup
- Margarine, diet	1/4 cup	1/4 cup
Baking powder biscuit, prepared with vegetable oil	1/4 cup	1/4 cup
- Apple	1 medium	1 medium
- Tea, unsweetened	1 cup	1 cup

Dinner		
- Pork stir-fry with vegetables		
Pork cutlet	2 oz	2 oz
Peanut oil	1 tsp	1 tsp
Soy sauce, low sodium	1 tsp	1 tsp
Broccoli	½ cup	½ cup
Carrots	1 cup	½ cup
Mushrooms	1/4 cup	½ cup
- Steamed white rice	1 cup	½ cup
- Tea, unsweetened	1 cup	1 cup
Snack		
- Almond cookies	2 cookies	-
- Milk 1%, lowfat	3/4 cup	3/4 cup

1,600 Calories	1,200 Calories
Calories....................................1,609	Calories....................................1,220
Total carbohydrate, % kcals...........56	Total Carbohydrates, % kcals........55
Total fat, % kcals...........................27	Total fat, % kcals...........................27
*Sodium, mg.............................1,296	*Sodium, mg............................1,043
Saturated fat, % kcals........8	Saturated fat, % kcals.......................8
Cholesterol, mg.............148	Cholesterol, mg...........................117
Protein, % kcals..............20	Protein, % kcals.......................... 21

1,600: 100% RDA met for all nutrients except zinc 95%, iron 87%, and calcium 93%

1,200: 100% RDA met for all nutrients except vitamin E 75%, calcium 84%, magnesium 98%, iron 66%, and zinc 77%.

*No salt added in recipe preparation or as seasoning. Consume at least 32 ounces of water.

Mexican American Cuisine - Reduced Calorie		
Breakfast	**1,600 Calories**	**1,200 Calories**
- Cantaloupe	1cup	½ cup
- Farina, prepared with 1%, lowfat milk	½ cup	½ cup
- White bread	1 slice	1 slice
- Margarine	1 tsp	1 tsp
- Jelly	1 tsp	1 tsp
- Orange juice	1 ½ cup	3/4 cup
- Milk, 1%, lowfat	½ cup	½ cup
Lunch		
- Beef enchilada:		
Tortilla, corn	2 tortillas	2 tortillas
Lean roast beef	2 ½ oz	2 oz
Vegetable oil	2/3 tsp	2/3 tsp
Onion	1 T	1 T
Tomato	4 T	4 T
Lettuce	½ cup	½ cup
Chili peppers'	2 tsp	2 tsp
Refried beans, prepared with vegetable oil	1/4 cup	1/4 cup

- Carrots - Celery - Milk, 1%, low fat - Water	5 sticks 6 sticks ½ cup -	5 sticks 6 sticks - 1 cup
Dinner - Chicken taco: Tortilla, corn Chicken breast, without skin Vegetable oil Cheddar cheese, lowfat and low sodium Guacamole Salsa - Corn, seasoned with margarine - Spanish rice without meat' - Banana - Coffee - Milk, 1%	 1 tortilla 2 oz 2/3 tsp 1 oz 2 T 1 T ½ cup ½ cup 1 large 1 cup 1 oz	 1 tortilla 1 oz 2/3 tsp ½ oz 1 T 1 T ½ cup ½ cup ½ large ½ cup 1 oz

Calories....................................1,638
Total carbohydrate, % kcals...........56
Total fat, % kcals...........................27
*Sodium, mg.............................1,616
Saturated fat, % kcals........9
Cholesterol, mg.............143
Protein, % kcals..............20

Calories..................................1,239
Total Carbohydrates, % kcals........58
Total fat, % kcals...........................26
*Sodium, mg...........................1,364
Saturated fat, % kcals......................8
Cholesterol, mg............................91
Protein, % kcals.......................... 19

1,600: 100% RDA met for all nutrients except vitamin E 97% and zinc 84%.
1,200: 100% RDA met for all nutrients except vitamin E 71%, vitamin B_1 & B_3 91%, vitamin B_2 & iron 90%, and calcium 92%.
*No salt added in recipe preparation or as seasoning. Consume at least 32 ounces of water.

Lacto-Ovo Vegetarian Cuisine - Reduced Calorie		
Breakfast	**1,600 Calories**	**1,200 Calories**
- Orange	1 medium	1 medium
-Pancakes, made with 1% lowfat milk and eggs white	3 4" circles -	1 4" circles -
- Pancake syrup	2 T	1 T
- Margarine, Diet	1 ½ tsp	1 ½ tsp
- Milk, 1%, lowfat	1 cup	½ cup
- Coffee	1 cup	1 cup
- Milk, 1%, lowfat	1 oz	1 oz

Lunch		
-Vegetable soup, canned, low sodium	1 cup	½ cup
-Bagel	1 medium	½ medium
- Processed american cheese, lowfat	3/4 oz	-
- Spinach salad:		
Spinach	1 cup	1 cup
Mushrooms	½ cup	½ cup
- Salad dressing, regular calorie	2 tsp	2 tsp
- Apple	1 medium	1 medium
- Iced tea, unsweetened	1 cup	1 cup
Dinner		
- Omelette:		
Egg whites	4 large eggs	4 large eggs
Green pepper	2 T	2 T
Onion	2 T	2 T
Mozzarella cheese, made from part skim milk, low sodium	1 oz	½ oz
Vegetable oil	1 T	½ T
- Brown rice, seasoned with Margarine,	½ cup	½ cup
diet	½ cup	½ tsp
- Carrots, seasoned with Margarine, diet	½ tsp	½ cup
- Whole wheat bread	1 slice	1 slice
- Margarine, diet	1 tsp	1 tsp
- Fig bar cookie	1 bar	1 bar
- Tea	1 cup	1 cup
- Honey	1 tsp	1 tsp
- Milk, 1%, lowfat	3/4 cup	3/4 cup

Calories....................................1,650	Calories....................................1,205
Total carbohydrate, % kcals...........56	Total Carbohydrates, % kcals........60
Total fat, % kcals...........................27	Total fat, % kcals...........................25
*Sodium, mg............................1,829	*Sodium, mg...........................1,335
Saturated fat, % kcals......................8	Saturated fat, % kcals......................7
Cholesterol, mg..............................82	Cholesterol, mg..............................44
Protein, % kcals............................19	Protein, % kcals.............................18

1,600: 100% RDA met for all nutrients except vitamin E 92%, vitamin B_3 97%, vitamin B_6 67%, iron 73%, and zinc68%.

1,200: 100% RDA met for all nutrients except vitamin E 75%, vitamin B_1 92%, vitamin B_3, 69%, vitamin B_6 59%, iron 54%, and zinc 46%.

*No salt added in recipe preparation or as seasoning. Consume at least 32 ounces of water.

Source: *NIH Publication #00-4084, October 2000*

APPENDIX XI

CALORIES, FAT, AND CHOLESTEROL IN FAST FOODS

	Calories	Fat (g)	Cholesterol (mg)
Arby's			
Roast Beef, reg	350	15	39
Roast Beef, Jr	218	8	20
Roast Beef, super	501	22	40
Roast Beef, deluxe	486	23	59
Beef'n Cheddar	490	21	51
Chicken Breast Sandwich	592	27	57
Potato Cakes, 2	201	14	1
French Fries	211	8	6
Bac'n Cheddar Deluxe	561	34	78
Hot Ham & Cheese	353	13	50
Turkey Deluxe	375	17	39
Baked Potato, plain	290	1	0
Superstuffed Potato, Deluxe	648	38	72
Roasted Chicken Breast	254	7	200
Chicken Salad Sandwich	386	20	30
Tossed Salad, plain	44	0	0
Vanilla Shake	295	30	30
Chocolate Shake	384	32	32
Burger King			
Whopper	640	41	94
Whopper, with cheese	723	48	117
Whopper Junior	370	17	41
Whopper Junior, cheese	420	20	52
Hamburger	275	12	37
Cheeseburger	317	15	48

Bacon Double Cheeseburger	510	31	104
French Fries, reg	227	13	14
Onion Rings, reg	274	16	0
Apple Pie	305	12	4
Whaler Fish Sandwich	488	227	84
Whaler, with cheese	530	30	95
Chicken Sandwich	688	40	82
Chicken Tenders	204	10	47
Breakfast Croissanwich			
Bacon, Egg, Cheese	355	24	249
Burger King (cont'd)			
Sausage, Egg, Cheese	538	41	293
Ham, Egg Cheese	335	20	262
Scrambled Egg Platter	468	30	370
Scrambled Egg Platter & Sausage	702	52	420
French Toast Sticks	469	30	73
Salad, plain	390	20	-
Danish Apple Pie	357	13	6
Kentucky Fried Chicken			
Wing, original recipe	181	12	67
Wing, extra crispy	218	16	63
Breast, original recipe	276	17	96
Breast, extra crispy	354	24	66
Drumstick, original recipe	147	9	81
Drumstick, extra crispy	173	11	65
Thigh, original recipe	278	19	122
Thigh, extra crispy	371	26	121
Kentucky Nuggets, 1	46	3	12
Kentucky Fries	268	13	2
Mashed Potatoes & Gravy	62	1	1
Buttermilk, Biscuit	269	14	1
McDonald's			
Chicken McNuggets	323	21	73
Hamburger	263	11	29
Cheeseburger	328	16	41
Quarter Pounder	427	24	81
Quarter Pounder, cheese	525	32	107
Big Mac	570	35	83

Filet-O-Fish	435	26	45
Mc D.L.T.	680	44	101
French Fries	220	12	9
Biscuit, Sausage, Egg	585	40	285
Biscuit, Bacon, Egg, Cheese	483	32	263
Sausage McMuffin	427	26	59
Sausage McMuffin, Egg	517	33	287
Egg McMuffin	340	16	259
Hot Cakes, butter, syrup	500	10	47
Scrambled Eggs	180	13	514
Sausage	210	19	39
English Muffin, butter	186	5	15
Hash Brown Potatoes	125	7	7
Strawberry Sundae	320	9	25
Hot Fudge Sundae	357	11	27
Caramel Sundae	361	10	31
Apple Pie	253	14	12
Cherry Pie	260	14	13
McDonaldland Cookies	308	11	10
Chocolate Chip Cookies	342	16	18
Chef's Salad	220	13	125
Shrimp Salad	99	3	187
Garden Salad	90	6	110
French Dressing, 1 packet	228	10	1
House Dressing, 1 packet	326	17	7
Blue Cheese Dressing, 1 packet	342	17	16
Vanilla Shake	352	8	31
Chocolate Shake	383	9	30

APPENDIX XII

NUTRIENT VALUES OF ENERGY BARS

BAR	CALORIES	FAT	SATURATED FAT	PRICE, $	COST PER 100 CALORIES, $
Zone Perfect	210	7	3	1.59	0.75
SlimFast Meal Bar	220	6	4	1.19	0.99
EAS Advantage Bar	220	6	3	2.19	0.99
Oneway Energy Bar	170	6	3	1.99	1.17
Luna	180	4.5	2.5	1.59	0.88
Balance Gold Triple Layer Energy Bar	210	7	4	1.53	0.73
Snickers Marathon	220	7	1.5	1.65	0.75
PowerBar	240	3.5	0.5	1.39	0.58
SlimFast	200	8	4	2.19	1.10
Clif Bar	250	6	1.5	1.49	0.60
Myoplex Lite Nutrition Bar	190	3.5	2.5	0.85	0.45
Atkins Advantage	220	10	6	2.49	1.13

APPENDIX XIII

CALORIES, FAT, AND CHOLESTEROL CONTENT OF SELECTED FOODS

Item	Portion	Calories	Fat g	Cholesterol mg
BEVERAGES:				
Alcoholic				
Beer				
Regular	12 fl. oz.	146	0.0	0
Light, Budweiser	12 fl. oz.	110	0.0	0
Champagne	6 fl. oz.	135	0.0	0
Gin, 80 proof	1-1/2 fl. oz.	103	0.0	0
Pina colada	6 fl. oz.	262	2.7	0
Rum, 80 proof	1-1/2 fl. oz.	103	0.0	0
Sherry, medium	6 fl. oz.	210	0.0	0
Vodka, 80 proof	1-1/2 fl. oz.	103	0.0	0
Whiskey, 80 proof	1-1/2 fl. oz.	103	0.0	0
Wine, dessert (18.8% alcohol)				
Dry	6 fl. oz.	224	0.0	0
Sweet	6 fl. oz.	272	0.0	0
BEVERAGES:				
Nonalcoholic				
Coca-Cola	12 fl. oz.	140	0.0	0
Coffee, regular brewed	6 fl. oz.	4	0.0	0
Coffee, Instant	6 fl. oz.	11	0.0	0
Coffee, Decaffeinated	6 fl. oz.	4	0.0	0
Fruit punch, canned Juice	1 cup	117	0.0	0
Apple, canned or bottled	1/2 cup	58	0.1	0
Blackberry, unsweetened, canned	1/2 cup	45	0.7	0
Cranberry	1/2 cup	75	0.1	0
Cranberry/apple, w/Vit. C	1/2 cup	82	0.0	0

Grape, canned or bottled	1/2 cup	77	0.1	0
Grape, sparkling Red, Welch's	6 fl. oz.	117	0.0	0
Grapefruit, canned				
Unsweetened	1/2 cup	47	0.1	0
Sweetened	1/2 cup	58	0.1	0
Orange, fresh	1/2 cup	56	0.2	0
Orange/grape canned	1/2 cup	53	0.1	0
Pineapple/grapefruit	1/2 cup	67	0.0	0
Pineapple/orange	1/2 cup	67	0.1	0
Pineapple, unsweetened,				
Canned	1/2 cup	70	0.1	0
Prune, canned or bottled	1/2 cup	91	0.0	0
Tomato, regular				
Canned/bottled	1/2 cup	21	0.1	0
Vegetable, Cocktail,				
Canned V-8, no salt	1/2 cup	23	0.1	0
Kool-Aid, cherry	1 cup	88	0.0	0
Lemonade,				
Regular, frozen, dilute	1 cup	99	0.0	0
Pink, prepared	1 cup	94	0.0	0
Nectar, canned				
Apricot	1/2 cup	70	0.1	0
Peach, 40% Fruit	1/2 cup	67	0.2	0
Seltzer, unsweetened	12 fl. oz.	0	0.0	0
Soda				
Club	12 fl. oz.	0	0.0	0
Orange	12 fl. oz.	170	0.0	0
Tang, orange, prepared	1 cup	119	0.0	0
Tea, brewed	6 fl. oz.	2	0.0	0
Tea, instant, prepared	6 fl. oz.	2	0.0	0
Quinine water	12 fl. oz.	121	0.0	0
BREADS AND BREADSTUFFS				
Bagels				
Plain-Lenders	1	190	2.0	5
Sara Lee	1	210	1.0	-
Biscuits				
Buttermilk	1	60	1.5	-
Breads				

7 Grain	1 slice	80	0.4	3
Brown, Boston, canned	1 slice	93	0.5	0
French				
Du Jour	1 slice	70	1.0	0
Garlic	1 slice	111	4.3	1
Pita				
Plain	1 slice	147	1.1	0
Pumpernickel	1 slice	76	0.4	0
Raisin	1 slice	66	0.7	1
Wheat				
Regular	1 slice	61	0.8	1
Pepperidge Farm	1 slice	95	1.5	-
White				
Wonder	1 slice	60	1.0	0
Breads, Sweetened				
Coffeecake	2 oz.	198	8.9	48
Danish				
Apple	1	335	15.9	19
Cheese	1	353	24.6	20
Donut	1	156	7.4	24
English Muffins				
Plain	1	182	3.6	32
Cinnamon Raisin-Chip	1	150	2.0	-
Pepperidge Farm	1	130	1.4	0
Thomas'	1	130	1.4	0
Rolls				
Pillsbury	1	95	5.0	-
Croissant				
Regular	1	272	17.3	47
Hamburger bun	1	136	3.4	13
Hot dog bun	1	136	3.4	13
BREAKFAST FOODS				
Cereal				
All Bran, Kellogg's	1/3 cup	69	1.0	0
Apple Jacks	1 cup	110	0.1	0
Cherrios, plain	1 cup	89	1.5	0
Honey Nut	1 cup	125	0.7	0
Cinnamon Toast Crunch	1 cup	160	4.0	0

Corn Flakes, Kellogg's				
Plain	1 cup	88	0.1	0
Sugar Frosted	1 cup	133	0.1	0
Farina, cooked	1 cup	116	0.2	0
Granola				
Cinnamon/raisin	1/2 cup	160	5.6	0
Grape-nuts	1/3 cup	135	0.2	0
Oat Bran O's				
Plain, Healthy Valley	1 cup	120	2.7	0
Fruit-n-Nut	1 cup	120	2.7	0
Oatmeal, cooked	1 cup	145	2.3	0
Oatmeal, instant	1 cup	94	2.0	0
Rice, puffed	1 cup	114	0.1	0
Rice Krispies	1 cup	112	0.2	0
Special K, Kellogg's	1 cup	83	0.1	0
Sugar Frosted Flakes, Kellogg's	1 cup	133	0.1	0
Wheaties	1 cup	99	0.5	0
Pancakes				
Blueberry, Aunt Jemima	2	136	1.0	-
Buttermilk	2	329	10.7	108
Prepared				
Plain	2 (4" ea.)	316	10.9	117
Mix, Aunt Jemima	1 oz.	61	2.3	-
Waffles				
Apple cinnamon Aunt Jemima	1	90	3.0	-
Belgian, frozen	1 (1.5 oz.)	120	4.0	5
CANDY				
Almond Joy	1.76 oz. Bar	142	7.9	-
Chocolate-coated	1 oz.	161	12.4	0
Sugar-coated	1 oz.	129	5.3	0
Baby Ruth	1.8 oz. Bar	145	6.1	0
Chocolate bar, plain				
Hershey	1 oz.	153	8.8	7
Nestle's	1 oz.	149	7.9	6
Chocolate bar w/nuts				
w/almonds, Cadbury	1 oz.	153	8.9	-
Hershey	1 oz.	159	10	8
Nestle's Crunch	1 oz.	149	7.9	6

COOKIES				
Brownie, w/o nuts				
Regular	1	243	10.1	10
Large, Hostess	1	243	9.6	17
Brownie w/nuts				
Regular	1	263	16.4	81
Fudge-n-Nut, Almost Home	1.2 oz.	160	7.0	-
Chocolate Chip				
Homemade	1	69	4.6	7
Pepperidge Farm	1	50	2.7	-
Gingersnap, small	1	36	1.3	3
CRACKERS				
Cheese Nips	1 oz.	132	5.7	-
Cheese & peanut butter	1 oz.	132	5.7	-
Nabisco	1/2 oz.	120	2.0	0
Triscuit	1 oz.	142	4.7	0
Wheat Thins, regular	1 oz.	142	6.0	0
DAIRY & DAIRY PRODUCTS				
Spread				
Cheese Whiz, Kraft	1 oz.	77	5.8	18
Swiss				
Regular	1 oz.	107	7.8	26
Kraft	1 oz.	92	7.0	23
Swiss, Lite				
Lifetime, non-fat	1 oz.	40	0.0	3
Weight Watchers, skim, semisoft	1 oz.	80	5.2	-
Milk & Milk Beverages				
Buttermilk, whole	1 cup	98	2.1	10
Condensed, sweetened, canned	2 tbl.	123	3.3	13
Cream, Half & Half	2 tbl.	39	3.5	11
Cream, heavy				
Whipped	2 tbl.	51	5.5	20
Unwhipped	2 tbl.	103	11.0	41
Cream, light (coffee or table)	1 tbl.	29	2.9	10
Cream, light (whipping)				

Whipped	2 tbl.	44	4.6	17
Unwhipped	2 tbl.	87	9.2	33
Cream, sour	2 tbl.	62	6.0	13
Half & Half	2 tbl.	41	3.6	11
Milk, chocolate, whole	1 cup	208	8.5	30
Milk, whole, 3.3% fat	1 cup	149	8.1	34
Milk, Low-fat				
1% fat	1 cup	102	2.5	10
2% fat	1 cup	122	4.7	20
Milk, skim	1 cup	86	0.4	5
Milk, non-fat				
Dry	1/4 cup	109	0.2	6
Instant, dry, Carnation	1 cup	260	0.5	13
Milkshake				
Chocolate	1 cup	282	6.4	24
Thick, frost,	1 cup	622	27.6	-
Quik, Nestle's				
Chocolate	2 tbl.	36	0.5	0
Strawberry	2 tbl.	41	0.0	0
Yogurt				
Plain				
Regular	1 cup	138	7.4	30
Low-fat	1 cup	143	3.5	14
Non-fat	1 cup	127	0.4	5
Flavored				
Coffee or vanilla, low-fat	1 cup	193	2.8	11
Fruit varieties, low-fat	1 cup	225	2.6	9
DESSERTS				
Angel Food				
Banana, Sara Lee	2 oz.	200	7.8	-
Carrot				
Homemade, prepared	2 oz.	203	11.9	32
Pepperidge Farm	2 oz.	204	11.6	-
Cheesecake, homemade				
Regular	2 oz.	188	13.7	64
Cheesecake, frozen	2 oz.	167	10.9	-
Chocolate, Commercial				
Loaf, nonfat, Entenmann's	2 oz.	140	0.0	0
light homemade fruit cake	2 oz.	221	9.4	0
German chocolate layer	2 oz.	222	12.3	-
Puddings				
Rice, w/raisins	1/2 cup	193	4.0	15

Tapioca	1/2 cup	111	4.1	80
Vanilla, instant prepared, from mix, Jello	1/2 cup	76	2.0	-
Other Desserts				
Baklava, homemade	1 oz.	112	8.2	20
Eclair				
Whipped cream filling & Chocolate icing	1	296	25.0	-
Trifle, chocolate	1	69	1.5	1
EGGS, EGG DISHES & EGG SUBSTITUTES				
Eggs				
White only, fresh, raw	1	16	0.0	0
Yolk only, fresh raw	1	61	5.2	218
Fried	1	54	6.8	207
Hard cooked	1	78	5.3	213
Poached, in salt water	1	75	5.0	212
Scrambled	1	103	7.6	218
Soft cooked	1	78	5.3	213
Egg Substitutes				
Egg Beaters, Fleischmann's	1/4 cup	30	0.0	0
FAST FOODS				
Arby's				
Apple turnover	1 serv.	310	21.0	0
Chicken breast				
Roasted	1 serv.	254	7.0	196
Sandwich	1 serv.	592	27.0	57
Kentucky Fried Chicken				
Bake bean	1 serv.	105	1.2	0
Bread, original, side order	1	276	17.3	96
Breast, center				
Original	1 serv.	257	13.7	93
Light/Crispy	1	220	11.9	93
Extra-crispy	1 serv.	353	20.9	93
Chicken nuggets	1 serv.	46	2.9	12
Coleslaw	1 serv.	103	5.7	4
Corn-on-the-cob	1 serv.	176	3.1	0
Drumstick				

Light/Crispy	1 serv.	121	7.0	95
Extra-crispy	1 serv.	173	3.1	95
French Fries	1 serv.	268	12.8	2
Gravy, Chicken	1 serv.	59	3.7	2
Potatoes, Mashed	1 serv.	59	0.6	0
Roll	1 serv.	269	13.6	-
Side Breast, extra-crispy	1 serv.	354	23.7	66
Thigh				
Original	1 serv.	278	19.2	122
Light/Crispy	1 serv.	246	16.7	-
Extra-crispy	1 serv.	371	26.3	121
Wing				
Original	1 serv.	181	12.3	67
Extra-crispy	1 serv.	218	15.6	63
McDonalds				
Big Mac	1 serv.	570	35.0	83
Biscuit				
with spread	1 serv.	287	18.2	9
with bacon/egg/cheese	1 serv.	483	31.5	262
with sausage	1 serv.	467	30.9	48
with sausage/egg	1 serv.	585	39.7	285
Danish				
Apple	1 serv.	389	17.9	26
Cheese, iced	1 serv.	395	21.7	48
Cheeseburger	1 serv.	315	15.8	40
Chicken McNuggetts	4 oz.	323	21.3	73
Cookies				
Chocolaty chip	1 serv.	337	16.0	18
McDonaldland	1 serv.	309	10.8	10
Dressings				
French, reduced calorie	1/2 oz.	40	1.9	0
Egg McMuffin	1 serv.	337	15.5	257
Filet-o-Fish	1 serv.	432	25.6	45
French fries				
Regular	1 serv.	220	11.4	9
Large	1 serv.	400	21.6	16
Hamburger	1 serv.	264	11.3	29
Ice cream cone	1 serv.	182	5.1	23
McChicken sandwich	1 serv.	490	28.6	43
McD.L.T.	1 serv.	681	43.9	101
McLean deluxe	1 serv.	320	10.0	60
Muffin				
Apple bran	1 serv.	190	0	0.0

English Muffin w/butter	1 serv.	186	5.3	15
Pancake w/butter & syrup	1 serv.	501	10.3	47
Pie				
Apple	1 serv.	253	14.2	13
Cherry	1 serv.	257	13.5	13
Potatoes, hash brown	1 serv.	125	7.0	50.4
Sausage	1 serv.	206	18.3	38
Sausage McMuffin				
Regular	1 serv.	423	26.0	58
With egg	1 serv.	513	32.6	285
Scrambled Eggs	1 serv.	180	13.0	514
Shake				
Chocolate	1 serv.	381	8.7	29
Strawberry	1 serv.	363	8.7	32
Vanilla	1 serv.	352	8.4	32
Taco Bell				
Burrito				
Bean	1 serv.	340	11.7	-
Beef	1 serv.	464	20.9	-
Combination	1 serv.	403	15.9	-
Enchirito	1 serv.	449	20.6	-
Pintos 'N' Cheese	1 serv.	167	5.0	-
Taco	1 serv.	183	7.9	-
Tostada				
Regular	1 serv.	177	5.9	-
Beefy	1 serv.	289	14.9	-
FATS AND OILS				
Butter				
Stick	1 tb.	102	11.5	31
Whipped	1 tb.	68	7.7	21
Butter, imitation				
Butter buds, dry powder	1 tb.	18	0.0	1
Butter buds, prepared	1 tb.	6	0.0	0
Molly McButter	1 tb.	24	0.0	0
Chicken Fat	1 tb.	115	12.8	11
Margarine				
Regular	1 tb.	101	11.4	0
Fleishchmann's	1 tb.	100	11.2	-
Mrs. Filbert's, 100% veg.	1 tb.	100	11	0

Mazola	1 tb.	101	11.2	0
Parkay Spread, 70% veg.	1 tb.	88	9.7	0
Promise Stick	1 tb.	90	10.0	0
Promise, soft	1 tb.	100	11.2	0
Margarine, light or diet, stick	1 tb.	50	5.6	0
Fleischmann's, Extra light	1 tb.	50	6.0	0
Fleischmann's, light	1 tb.	81	8.1	0
Oil, all types	1 tb.	121	13.6	0
Pam, spray	1 spray	2	0.2	0
FISH AND SHELLFISH				
Abalone, raw	3 oz.	89	0.6	72
Bass				
Black Sea, raw	3 oz.	97	3.1	58
Stripped, raw	3 oz.	82	2.0	68
Crab				
Blue, canned, drained	3 oz.	84	1.0	76
Blue, cooked	3 oz.	87	1.5	85
Fish sticks, frozen, cooked	1	76	3.4	31
Fish cake, frozen, cooked	3 oz.	231	10.4	95
Halibut, cooked	3 oz.	119	2.5	35
Mackerel, Atlantic, cooked	3 oz.	223	15.1	64
Monkfish, raw	3 oz.	65	1.3	21
Perch, ocean				
Raw	3 oz.	80	1.4	36
Cooked	3 oz.	103	1.8	46
Rockfish, cooked	3 oz.	103	1.7	37
Salmon				
Atlantic, raw	3 oz.	121	5.4	47
Pink, canned	3 oz.	118	5.1	-
Smoked (Lox)	3 oz.	100	3.7	20
Sockeye, canned	3 oz.	130	6.2	37
Sardine				
Atlantic, canned in oil	3 1/2 oz.	200	11.0	17
Shrimp				
Fried, breaded	3 oz.	206	10.4	151
Steamed, large	3 oz.	84	0.9	151
Sole				
Raw	3 oz.	77	1.0	41
Cooked	3 oz.	100	1.3	58
Tuna, canned				
Light, in oil, drained	3 oz.	225	19.1	36
Light, in water drained	3 oz.	90	1.5	36

FRUITS				
Apples				
Fresh	1	81	0.0	0
Dried	1	19	0.0	0
Applesauce				
Canned, unsweetened	1/2 cup	52	0.0	0
Canned, sweetened	1/2 cup	97	0.0	0
Apricots				
Fresh	1	18	0.0	0
Canned w/skin, heavy syrup	1/2 cup	114	0.0	0
Dried, uncooked	1	17	0.0	0
Avocado, fresh				
California	1	306	29.8	0
Florida	1	339	26.7	0
Banana, fresh	1	109	0.0	0
Blackberries				
Fresh	1/2 cup	37	0.0	0
Frozen, unsweetened, Not thawed	1/2 cup	48	0.0	0
Blueberries				
Fresh	1/2 cup	41	0.0	0
Frozen, unsweetened	2 cup	42	0.0	0
Cantaloupe, fresh	1/4 cup	45	0.0	0
Cherries, fresh				
Sour, red w/o pits	1/2 cup	39	0.0	0
Sweet	1/2 cup	52	0.0	0
Cherries, canned				
Sour, red, water, packed	1/2 cup	44	0.0	0
Sour, red, heavy syrup	1/2 cup	127	0.0	0
Sweet, water-packed	1/2 cup	62	0.0	0
Sweet, heavy syrup	1/2 cup	107	0.2	0
Cherries, Maraschino	1/2 cup	162	0.0	0
Coconut				
Fresh	1 whole	1,349	128	0
Shredded, dried, sweetened	1 1/2 cup	232	16.4	0
Crabapples, fresh	1 each	23	0.0	0
Cranberries, fresh	1/2 cup	23	0.0	0
Cranberry sauce, canned, sweetened	1/2 cup	209	0.0	0

Currants, fresh				
Black, European	1/2 cup	35	0.0	0
Red or white	1/2 cup	31	0.0	0
Figs				
Fresh, medium	1	37	0.0	0
Dried	1	48	0.0	0
Canned, light syrup	1/2 cup	87	0.0	0
Fruit Cocktail, canned				
Juice packed	1/2 cup	57	0.0	0
In heavy syrup	1/2 cup	93	0.0	0
Fruit Salad, canned				
Water packed	1/2 cup	37	0.0	0
Heavy syrup	1/2 cup	93	0.0	0
Grapefruit				
fresh	1	77	0.0	0
Canned, sweetened	1/2 cup	76	0.0	0
Grapes, fresh				
Concord	1/2 cup	29	0.0	0
Emperor	1/2 cup	57	0.0	0
Thompson	1/2 cup	57	0.0	0
Guavas, common fresh	1	41	0.0	0
Honeydew, fresh cubed	1/2 cup	30	0.0	0
Kiwi fruit	1	44	0.0	0
Kumquat, fresh	1	12	0.0	0
Lemons, fresh				
with peel	1	22	0.0	0
without peel	1	16	0.0	0
Plum				
fresh	1	35	0.0	0
purple, canned, in heavy syrup	1/2 cup	115	0.0	0
Pomegranate pulp, fresh	1	104	0.0	0
Prunes				
Dried, uncooked	1 med	20	0.0	0
Cooked, no sugar	1/2 cup	134	0.0	0
Quince, fresh	1	52	0.0	0
Raisins				
Black	1/2 cup	217	0.0	0
Golden	1/2 cup	219	0.0	0
Raspberries				
Black, fresh	1/2 cup	33	0.0	0
Red, fresh	1/2 cup	30	0.0	0
Red, frozen, sweetened	1/2 cup	129	0.0	0
Rhubarb, cooked, added				

sugar	1/2 cup	157	0.0	0
Strawberries				
Fresh	1 cup	45	0.0	0
Frozen, unsweetened	1 cup	52	0.0	0
Tangerines	1	38	0.0	0
Watermelon, fresh, diced	1/2 cup	26	0.0	0
ICE CREAM, FROZEN YOGURT AND NON-DAIRY FROZEN DESSERTS				
Ice Cream				
Chocolate	1/2 cup	155	7.2	19
Chocolate cup, Breyers	5 oz.	160	8.0	-
Strawberry	1/2 cup	116	5.0	16
Vanilla				
10% fat, regular	1/2 cup	134	7.2	30
16% fat, rich	1/2 cup	175	11.8	44
Frozen Yogurt				
Low-fat, Colombo	4 fl. oz.	99	2.0	10
Non-fat				
Colombo	4 fl. oz.	95	0.0	0
TCBY	4 fl. oz.	110	1.0	5
Sherbert, lemon	1/2 cup	104	0.9	0
Sorbet, strawberry	1/2 cup	71	0.3	0
MEAT				
Beef				
Brisket, flat, lean, braised	3 oz.	224	13.5	77
Chuck, Arm, lean, braised	3 oz.	196	8.5	86
Blade, lean, braised	3 oz.	230	13.0	90
Ground				
Extra-lean, boiled	3 oz. patty	218	13.9	71
Lean, broiled	3 oz. patty	231	15.7	74
Rib eye, lean, broiled	3 oz.	191	9.9	68
Round				
Bottom, lean, braised	3 oz.	189	8.2	82
Eye, lean, roasted	3 oz.	156	4.0	77
Tip, lean, roasted	3 oz.	162	6.4	69
Top, lean, broiled	3 oz.	162	5.3	71
Steak, flank, lean, broiled	3 oz.	207	12.7	60

Tenderloin, lean broiled	3 oz.	173	7.9	71
Lamb				
Chop				
Loin, broiled, lean only	3 oz.	160	6.0	44
Loin, broiled, lean & fat	3 oz.	305	25.0	85
Rib				
Cooked, lean only	3 oz.	200	11.0	77
Cooked, lean & fat	3 oz.	307	25.2	84
Shoulder				
Cooked, lean only	3 oz.	173	9.2	74
Cooked, lean & fat	3 oz.	290	23.0	78
Leg, lean, roasted	3 oz.	160	6.0	79
Ham				
Country style, cured, lean	3 oz.	173	10.9	46
Fresh				
Roasted, lean and fat	3 oz.	233	15.1	81
Loin, sirloin, raw lean only	3 oz.	128	5.7	54
Lean and fat	3 oz.	235	19.0	60
Pork				
Boston butt, roasted, lean only	3 oz.	233	15.1	81
Chop, lean, loin braised	3 oz.	230	12.0	56
Rib, lean, braised	3 oz.	230	12.0	0
Veal				
Cubed, for stew, braised, lean only	3 oz.	160	3.7	123
Cutlet, breaded	3 oz.	115	2.3	14
Leg, braised				
Lean only	3 oz.	173	4.3	115
Lean & fat	3 oz.	179	5.4	114
Prepared or Processed Meats				
Bacon, regular				
Canadian, broiled or fried, drained	1 slice	37	1.7	12
Cured, broiled or fried, drained	1 slice	43	3.7	6

Bacon Bits, imitation	3 oz.	264	25.1	0
Beef, Sizzlelean	2 strips	70	5.0	-
Breakfast strips,				
Sizzlelean	1 slice	49	3.9	-
Beef, corned				
Buddig, lean	1 slice	40	2.0	-
Canned	1 oz.	71	4.2	24
Cooked	1 oz.	71	5.4	28
Bologna				
Beef, Oscar Mayer	1 slice	72	6.7	13
Beef & Pork	2 oz.	179	16.0	31
Turkey, Louis Rich	1 slice	58	4.7	19
Chicken roll, light meat	2 oz.	90	4.2	28
Chicken, sliced Buddig	1 slice	60	4.0	-
Corn dog	1	460	18.9	79
Frankfurter				
Beef, Oscar Mayer	1	141	13.2	27
Pork & beef w/cheese	2 oz.	185	16.4	39
Ham Loaf, glazed	3 oz.	236	14.3	90
Ham, chopped, canned	3 oz.	203	16.0	42
Hot Dog				
Beef	1	176	16.0	34
Chicken	1	113	8.6	44
Pastrami				
Beef	2 oz.	198	16.5	53
Turkey	2 oz.	69	2.9	31
Pate				
Chicken liver, canned	3 oz.	171	11.1	-
Pepperoni, pork and beef	1 slice	27	2.4	4
Pork, cooked	3 oz.	256	21.9	51
Salami				
Beef	2 oz.	142	11.4	37
Pork, dry or hard	2 oz.	231	19.1	-
Sausage				
Brown 'n' Serve, Jones	1 link	100	10.0	-
Light, w/rice, Jones	1 link	70	5.5	-
NUTS, SEEDS & PEANUT BUTTER				
Almonds, raw, natural				
Blue Diamond	1 oz.	165	14.9	0
Beechnuts, shelled	1 oz.	163	14.2	0

Brazil nuts, dried	2 tb.	115	11.6	0
Cashews				
Dry roasted	2 tb.	98	7.9	0
Oil-roasted, Planters	1 tb.	170	14.0	0
Chestnut, fresh	2 tb.	39	0.4	0
Coconut				
Raw, not packed	2 tb.	35	3.4	0
Dried, sweetened shredded	1 tb.	29	2.1	0
Hazelnuts, shelled whole	2 tb.	107	10.6	0
Macadamia, dried	2 tb.	118	12.4	0
Mixed				
Oil-roasted, no peanuts	2 tb.	111	10.1	0
Roasted w/peanuts	2 tb.	110	10.0	0
Peanuts, roasted				
In shell	1 cup	209	17.7	0
with oil	1/2 cup	450	35.0	0
Dry roasted, Planters	1 oz.	160	13.9	-
Honey roasted, Planters	1 oz.	170	13.0	0
Peanut Butter				
Chunky	1 tb.	95	8.1	0
Smooth	1 tb.	95	8.3	0
Pecans, shelled, halves	2 tb.	90	9.1	0
Pine, pignolia	2 tb.	103	10.1	0
Pistachio, dry roasted	2 tb.	92	7.7	0
Poppy seeds	2 tb.	94	7.8	0
Pumpkin seed kernels, dry	2 tb.	93	7.9	0
Sesame seeds, dry, whole	2 tb.	103	8.9	0
Sunflower seeds	2 tb.	103	8.9	0
Trail mix, w/coconut	1 oz.	143	11.0	0
Walnuts, Black	2 tb.	95	8.8	0
Persian or English shelled, halves	2 tb.	80	7.7	0
PASTA & NOODLES				
Macaroni, regular Cooked	1 cup	197	0.9	0
Cooked, al dente	1 cup	155	0.6	0
Spirals, cooked	1 cup	189	0.9	0
Manicotti, cheese, stouffer's	8 oz.	234	10.9	34
Noodles, chow mein canned	1 cup	237	13.8	0
Noodles, egg, cooked	1 cup	213	2.4	53
Dry	2 oz.	216	2.4	54
Noodles, lasagna, cooked	1 cup	197	0.9	0
Spaghetti cooked	1 cup	155	0.6	0

Spaghetti twist, w/sauce, Buitoni	15 oz. can	300	8.0	0
POULTRY				
Chicken				
Breast, baked or broiled				
no skin	1/2 breast	142	3.0	73
with skin	1/2 breast	193	7.6	82
Breast, fried, no skin, boneless	1/2 breast	161	4.1	78
with skin	1/2 breast	338	17.0	111
Capon, w/skin, roasted	3 oz.	195	9.9	73
Fryer, dark meat, no skin				
Fried	3 oz.	203	9.9	82
Roasted	3 oz.	174	8.3	79
Stewed	3 oz.	163	7.6	75
Fryer, dark meat w/skin				
Floured, fried	3 oz.	242	14.2	78
Roasted	3 oz.	215	13.4	77
Stewed	3 oz.	198	12.5	70
Fryer, white meat, no skin				
Roasted	3 oz.	147	3.8	72
Stewed	3 oz.	135	3.4	65
Fryer, white meat w/skin				
Fried	3 oz.	163	4.7	77
Roasted	3 oz.	189	9.2	71
Stewed	3 oz.	171	8.5	63
Fryer, heart, simmered	3 oz.	157	6.7	206
Fryer, wing meat, w/skin				
Fried	3 oz.	276	18.5	67
Roasted	3 oz.	247	16.5	71
Stewed	1	100	6.7	28
Giblets, cooked	3 oz.	134	4.0	334
Gizzards, simmered	3 oz.	130	3.1	165
Leg, baked or broiled				
no skin, drum/thigh	1	178	7.8	87
with skin, drum/thigh	1	260	15.1	103
Leg, fried, w/skin	1	431	25.5	142
Liver, cooked	3 oz.	134	4.6	537
Roaster, meat only roasted	3 oz.	142	5.6	64
Poultry, Game				

Duck				
Domesticated, roasted	3 oz.	171	9.4	76
Pheasant, raw	3 oz.	113	3.1	-
Quail, raw (out)	3 oz.	114	3.9	-
Goose, domesticated				
liver, raw	1	124	4.0	550
Roasted, no skin	3 oz.	202	10.8	82
with skin	3 oz.	259	18.6	77
Turkey				
Light and dark, roasted,				
meat only, no skin	3 oz.	145	4.2	65
with skin	3 oz.	177	8.3	70
Breast, w/skin	3 oz.	161	6.3	63
Dark meat, cooked				
no skin	3 oz.	159	6.1	72
with skin	3 oz.	188	9.8	76
RICE AND GRAINS				
Rice				
Brown, cooked	1/2 cup	108	0.9	0
Cakes, Chico San				
Buckwheat, no salt	1	36	0.2	0
With millet, no salt	1	36	0.2	0
Plain, no salt	1	36	0.2	0
Mix, chicken, Rice-A-Roni,				
Prepared	1/2 cup	107	0.7	-
White, cooked	1/2 cup	132	0.3	-
White, long grain				
Instant cooked	1/2 cup	81	0.1	0
Minute Rice	2/3 cup	120	0.0	0
Wild Uncooked	1/2 cup	286	0.9	0
Wild Cooked	1/2 cup	83	0.3	0
Wild, long grain, Minute				
Rice, Cooked	1/2 cup	148	4.0	10
SALADS				
Beans, garbanzo, cooked,				
broiled and drained	2 tb.	34	0.5	0
Broccoli, raw, chopped	2 tb.	3	0.0	0
Carrots, raw, diced	2 tb.	7	0.0	0
Coleslaw, Regular, made				
w/mayonnaise	1/2 cup	41	1.6	5
Crouton	1	30	1.0	0

Cucumbers, raw, not pared	2 tb.	2	0.0	0
Lettuce	1 cup	7	0.1	0
Macaroni, made				
w/mayonnaise	1/2 cup	349	23.4	136
Mushrooms, raw	2 tb.	2	0.0	0
Onions, raw, chopped	2 tb.	8	0.0	0
Pasta w/seafood	1 cup	243	1.8	70
Peppers, green, raw, strips	1/2 cup	3	0.0	0
Tomatoes, fresh, chopped	2 tb.	5	0.0	0
SALAD DRESSINGS				
Blue Cheese, Kraft	1 tb.	76	7.6	4
Blue Cheese, low calorie				
Kraft	1 tb.	59	5.8	11
Wishbone	1 tb.	40	4.0	0
Blue Cheese, mix				
Good Season	1 tb.	3	0.0	0
Coleslaw, commercial	1 tb.	57	4.9	4
French Homemade	1 tb.	87	9.6	-
Kraft, Catalina	1 tb.	65	5.6	0
Kraft, regular	1 tb.	59	5.7	0
French, low-fat				
Kraft Free	1 tb.	20	0.0	0
Wishbone	1 tb.	2	0.0	0
Italian				
Bernstein's	1 tb.	32	1.0	0
Kraft, creamy	1 tb.	55	5.5	1
Kraft	1 tb.	73	7.7	0
Italian, low-calorie				
Good Season, zesty, light	1 tb.	25	0.0	0
Kraft	1 tb.	7	0.0	0
Wishbone	1 tb.	1	0.0	0
Italian, low-fat				
Kraft Free	1 tb.	6	0.0	0
No oil	1 tb.	8	0.0	0
Oil free, Kraft	1 tb.	4	0.0	0
Wishbone, creamy light	1 tb.	6	0.0	0
Mayonnaise				
Regular	1 tb.	99	10.9	8
Hellman's	1 tb.	98	10.8	10
Ranch, low-fat				
Kraft Free	1 tb.	16	0.0	0

Roka, reduced-calorie, Kraft	1 tb.	14	0.9	3
Russian	1 tb.	76	7.8	-
SNACKS				
Corn Chips				
Corn Snackers, Weight Watchers	1 oz.	121	4.0	-
Fritos	1 oz.	150	10.0	0
Black bean, garden	1 oz.	130	7.0	0
Doritos	1 oz.	140	6.0	0
Tostitos	1 oz.	140	8.0	0
Dips				
Avocado, Kraft	2 tb.	50	4.0	0
Blue cheese, Kraft, premium	2 tb.	45	4.0	10
Clam, Kraft	2 tb.	60	4.0	10
Guacamole	2 tb.	34	3.1	2
Onion, French, Kraft	2 tb.	60	4.0	0
Popcorn				
Air-popped	1 cup	23	0.3	0
Popped w/oil & salt	1 cup	41	2.0	0
Potato Chips				
Barbecue	1 oz.	152	9.4	0
Light, Pringles	1 oz.	130	6.0	0
Cape Cod	1 oz.	150	8.0	0
Eagle	1 oz.	150	10.0	0
Hawaiian	1 oz.	150	8.0	0
Pringles	1 oz.	160	11.0	0
Regular				
Lay's	1 oz.	150	10.0	0
Pringles	1 oz.	160	11.0	0
Ruffles	1 oz.	150	10.0	0
Pretzels				
Eagle	1 oz.	110	2.0	0
Mister Salty	1 oz.	109	1.1	0
Sticks, Mister Salty	10 sticks	101	0.0	0
No fat, thick, Snyder's	1 oz.	101	0.0	0
Soft commercial	1	145	0.4	0
Other Snacks				
Cheese Straws	1 oz.	128	8.4	-

Cheetos				
Crunchy	1 oz.	160	10.0	-
Light cheese snack	.9 oz.	120	6.0	-
Puffed balls	1 oz.	160	10.0	-
Corn nuts	1 oz.	129	4.3	0
Cracker Jacks	1 oz.	115	1.0	0
Fruit snacks, cherry,				
Grocer's choice	1 oz.	99	0.0	0
Fun Fruits, sunkist,	9 oz.	100	1.0	-
Funyuns	1 oz.	140	6.0	0
SOUPS				
Asparagus Cream of, canned				
Prepared w/water	1 cup	85	4.1	5
Prepared w/milk	1 cup	161	7.9	22
Beef bouillon				
Cubes dehydrated	1	6	0.1	-
Granules, Herb-Ox	1 pkg.	8	0.0	-
Beef consomme, canned				
w/water	1 cup	31	0.0	24
Beef Noodle				
Canned w/water	1 cup	83	3.1	5
Broth, chicken, low-fat	1 cup	22	0.0	0
Broth, chicken, Pritikin	1 cup	16	0.0	0
Chicken, cream of chicken				
and dumplings	1 cup	96	5.5	34
Chicken gumbo, Campbell				
Prepared	1 cup	55	1.2	-
Chicken Noodles				
Dehydrated w/water	1 cup	53	1.2	3
Chicken Rice				
Dehydrated w/water	1 cup	61	1.4	3
Clam Chowder,				
New England	1 cup	87	2.5	-
Consomme chicken,				
canned	1 cup	39	1.4	0
Mix, w/gelatin	1 pkt.	78	0.1	0
Corn chowder, homemade	1 cup	180	5.1	6
Lentil, homemade	1 cup	132	1.6	0
Minestrone, homemade	1 cup	113	1.7	2
Prepared, canned w/water	1 cup	82	2.5	2

Chunky, ready-to-serve	1 cup	127	2.8	5
Campbell	1 cup	92	2.4	-
Progresso	1 cup	30	1.8	2
Tabachnik	7.5 oz.	137	2.0	0
Dehydrated, prepared w/water	1 cup	79	1.7	3
Mushroom, cream of, canned, prepared w/water	1 cup	129	9.0	2
prepared w/milk	1 cup	203	13.6	20
with beef stock, prepared w/water	1 cup	85	4.0	7
Split pea, canned, prepared, w/water	1 cup	190	4.3	8
Tomato, canned				
prepared w/milk	1 cup	161	6.0	17
prepared w/water	1 cup	85	1.9	0
Tomato bisque, canned prepared w/water	1 cup	124	2.5	5
Tomato rice, canned, w/water	1 cup	119	2.7	2
Vegetable, vegetarian Campbell, prepared w/water	1 cup	78	1.2	0
Spices & Condiments				
Catsup				
Heinz	1 tb.	18	0.0	0
Del Monte	1 tb.	14	0.1	0
Heinz, low-salt	1 tb.	8	0.0	0
Olives				
Black, ripe, pitted, medium	2	9	0.9	0
Pickle sweet, whole	1 lg.	50	0.1	0
Pimento, canned solids & liquid	2 tb.	9	0.1	0
Shake 'N' Bake				
Chicken, BBQ, dry	1/2 oz.	53	1.1	0
Soy sauce	1 tb.	8	0.0	0
Vinegar				
Cider	2 tb.	4	0.0	0
Distilled, white	2 tb.	4	0.0	0
VEGETABLES AND BEANS				
Bean & Bean Products				

Baked, vegetarian Canned S&W	1/2 cup	115	1.0	0
Baked w/pork, canned Campbell	1/2 cup	120	1.5	9
Chickpeas, dried, boiled & Drained	1/2 cup	134	2.0	0
Kidney, dark red, canned w/solids & liquid	1/2 cup	109	0.0	0
Lentils, dried boiled and drained	1/2 cup	115	0.0	0
Lima, baby, frozen cooked, boiled & drained	1/2 cup	94	0.0	0
Lima, immature, dried, boiled and drained	1/2 cup	105	0.0	0
Lima, mature, dried, boiled and drained	1/2 cup	108	0.0	0
Mung, sprouted, seeds, raw	1/2 cup	16	0.0	0
Mung, sprouts, no seeds	1/2 cup	13	0.0	0
Pinto, cooked, boiled and drained	1/2 cup	117	0.0	0
Red, dried, boiled, drained	1/2 cup	112	0.0	0
Refried, canned, Old El Paso	1/2 cup	130	2.0	-
Refried, vegetarian Rosarita	1/2 cup	120	2.0	0
Soybeans, cooked boiled & drained	1/2 cup	149	7.7	0
Split peas, cooked	1/2 cup	115	0.0	0
Sprouts	1/2 cup	16	0.0	0
Tempeh, fermented Soybean product	1/2 cup	165	6.4	0
Tofu, raw, firm	1/2 cup	183	11.0	0
White, small, cooked	1/2 cup	127	0.6	0
Vegetables & Potatoes				
Alfalfa sprouts	1/2 cup	5	0.0	0
Artichokes, fresh	1	53	0.2	0
Artichoke hearts, boiled, drained canned	1/2 cup	37	0.0	0
Asparagus Canned, drained	1 each	3	0.0	0
Bamboo shoots, raw	1/2 cup	20	0.0	0
Beets, fresh, cooked	1	16	0.0	0
Beets, red, pickled, canned solids & liquid	2 tb.	18	0.0	0

Beets, pickled, canned, solids & liquids	1/2 cup	74	0.0	0
Broccoli, fresh w/cheese	1/2 cup	12	0.0	0
Birds Eye	5 oz.	110	5.0	-
Brussel sprouts, fresh, cooked	1/2 cup	30	0.0	0
Cabbage, Chinese	1/2 cup	5	0.0	0
Cabbage, red				
cooked	1/2 cup	16	0.0	0
raw	1/2 cup	9	0.0	0
Cabbage, white, raw	1/2 cup	8	0.0	0
Carrots, raw	1	31	0.0	0
Cauliflower, Cooked	1/2 cup	15	0.0	0
raw, florets	1/2 cup	19	0.0	0
Cauliflower, frozen, w/cheese, sauce, Birds Eye	4 oz.	127	8.6	-
Celery				
cooked	1/2 cup	13	0.0	0
fresh, stalk	1 each	6	0.0	0
Chinese, raw cabbage	1/2 cup	34	0.0	0
Collard greens (see Greens)				
Corn, sweet, fresh				
Yellow kernels	1/2 cup	90	0.0	0
White Kernels	1/2 cup	90	0.0	0
Corn, sweet, canned				
Cream style	1/2 cup	92	0.0	0
Corn on the cob	1 med.	80	0.0	0
Corn souffle	1 serv.	160	7.0	-
Cucumbers, whole, not pared	1	32	0.0	0
Eggplant, boiled, drained	1/2 cup	13	0.0	0
Endive, Belgian	1/2 cup	7	0.0	0
Escarole, raw	1/2 cup	4	0.0	0
Ginger root, raw	1/2 cup	33	0.0	0
Greens				
Collard, cooked, drained	1/2 cup	12	0.0	0
Mustard, boiled, drained	1/2 cup	10	0.0	0
Turnip				
Fresh, cooked	1/2 cup	14	0.0	0
Frozen, cooked	1/2 cup	25	0.0	0
Kale, cooked, leaves and stems	1/2 cup	21	0.0	0
Kohlrabi, thick, bulb only,				

cooked	1/2 cup	24	0.0	0
Leeks, bulb & lower leaf,				
cooked	1 serv.	76	0.0	0
Lettuce, raw				
Butterhead	1/2 cup	4	0.0	0
Crisphead, chopped	1/2 cup	4	0.0	0
Mixed, Italian, frozen	1/2 cup	25	0.0	0
Mushrooms				
Fresh, raw	1	4	0.0	0
Canned, solids & liquids	1/2 cup	15	0.0	0
Okra, cooked	1/2 cup	26	0.0	0
Onions, canned, french fried,				
Durkee	1/2 cup	176	0.0	0
Onion rings	1 oz.	276	0.0	0
Parsley, fresh raw	1/2 cup	10	0.0	0
Parsnips, boiled and diced	1/2 cup	63	0.0	0
Peas & carrots, frozen,				
boiled and drained	1/2 cup	38	0.0	0
Peas, Black Eye, cooked	1/2 cup	90	0.0	0
Peas, green, fresh cooked	1/2 cup	67	0.0	0
Peas, green, canned	1/2 cup	102	4.4	0
Le Sueur, Green Giant				
Peas, snow, cooked	1/2 cup	34	0.0	0
Peppers				
Bell, chopped	1/2 cup	19	0.0	0
Hot chili				
Green, chopped	1/2 cup	30	0.0	0
Red, chopped	1/2 cup	29	0.0	0
Pimiento, canned				
solids & liquid	1/2 cup	35	0.0	0
Potatoes, Fresh				
Baked w/skin	1	218	0.0	0
Boiled	1	116	0.0	0
Boiled, pared, diced				
or sliced	1/2 cup	67	0.0	0
French-fried, homemade	1/2 cup	90	4.7	0
Potatoes, frozen				
French fried				
Cottage fries,				
Birds Eye	4 oz.	171	7.1	0
Birds Eye	1	37	1.3	0
Light, Ore-Ida	3 oz.	90	2.0	0

Hashbrown, shredded, Ore-Ida	1/2 cup	57	0.0	0
Potatoes, sweet				
Boiled w/o skin, mashed	1/2 cup	172	0.0	0
Baked in skin	1	115	0.0	0
Yams, cooked, baked	1/2 cup	79	0.0	0
Rutabage, boiled sliced	1/2 cup	29	0.0	0
Scallions, raw	1/2 cup	16	0.0	0
Spinach, raw	1/2 cup	6	0.0	0
Squash, Acorn boiled, mashed	1/2 cup	42	0.0	0

APPENDIX XIV

CALORIC CONTENT OF ALCOHOLIC AND NONALCOHOLIC BEVERAGES

Drink Serving Sizes:						
1	cordial glass	= 2/3 oz		1	champagne glass	= 5 oz
1	brandy glass	= 1 oz		1	tumbler	= 8-12 oz
1	sherry glass	= 2 oz		1	mixing glass	= 12 oz
1	cocktail glass	= 3 oz		1	jigger	= 1 2 oz
1	burgundy glass	= 4 oz				

Distilled Spirits - Brandy, Bourbon, Cognac, Canadian Whisky, Gin, Rye, Scotch, and Tequila (per 1 jigger = 1 2 oz)

Proof	**Calories**	**Grams of Carbohydrates**	**Grams of Alcohol**
80	100	0	14
84	105	0	15
86	108	0	15 2
90	112	0	16
94	117	0	16 2
94.6	118	0	16 2
97	121	0	17
100	124	0	18

CALORIC CONTENT OF ALCOHOLIC BEVERAGES

Beverages	**Amount**	**Grams of Carbohydrate**	**Grams of Alcohol**	**Calories**
Liqueurs and Cordials	2/3 oz	4-10	4-7	50-80
Malt Liquors				
Ale, Beer, Stout	12 oz	14	13	151
Light Beer	12 oz	6	10	90
Near Beer	12 oz	12	2	60
Wines				
Sweet domestic	3.2 oz	8-14	13-15	140-165
sweet imported	3.2 oz	3-20	10 2 - 18	110-175
dry domestic	3.2 oz	2 -4	10-11	75-90
dry imported	3.2 oz	2 -3	8-14	60-110
Champagne	4 oz	4	12	98
Eggnog with Rum	4 oz (12 oz rum)	18	20	335

Beverage	**Amount**	**Calories**	**Carbohydrate (g)**
Liqueur and Brandy			
Kahlua	1 ½ oz	178	24
Apricot Brandy	1 ½ oz	99	9
Cognac	1 ½ oz	110	0
Mix Drinks			
Daiquiri	6 oz	325	12
Kahlua and Cream	6 oz	567	36
Martini	6 oz	383	1

CALORIE CONTENT OF NONALCOHOLIC BEVERAGES

Beverage Item	**Amount**	**Calories**	**Carbohydrate (g)**
Carbonated Soft Drinks – Regular			
Coca-Cola Classic®-small	16 oz	150	38
Coca-Cola Classic®-medium	21oz	210	55
Coca-Cola Classic®-large	32 oz	300	82
Sprite-small	16oz	140	37
Sprite-medium	21oz	210	53
Sprite-large	32oz	300	78
Carbonated Soft Drinks – Diet			
Diet Coke®-small	16 oz	1	0
Diet Coke®-medium	21 oz	2	0
Diet Coke®-large	32 oz	3	0
Diet Seven Up	12 oz	4	0
New Age Beverages-Regular			
Twister-Orange Peach	8 oz	120	29
Twister light-Orange Cranberry	8 oz	30	7
Arizona Ice Tea-Mucho Mango	8 oz	100	27
Arizona Ice Tea-ice tea	8 oz	95	25
Clearly Canadian-Wild Cherry	11 oz	120	31
Snapple-Fruit Punch	8 oz	120	29
Snapple-Orange-flavored tea	8 oz	110	27
Fruitopia-Raspberry Psychic Lemonade	8 oz	120	30
Nestea ice tea-Peach	32 oz	3	0

MILK, COFFEE, TEA

Beverage Item	Amount	Calories	Carbohydrate (g)
MILK			
Regular	8 oz	150	12
Low fat	8 oz	110	11
Skim	8 oz	80	12
COFFEE			
Black	8 oz	3	0
TEA			
Black	8 oz	1	0
Ice tea-unsweetened	16 oz	6	0
Ice tea-sweetened	16 oz	203	50

APPENDIX XV

FROZEN, MICROWAVE, AND REFRIGERATED FOODS

FOOD	AMOUNT	CALORIES TOTAL	CALORIES FAT
APPETIZERS			
Cocktail beef franks (Cohen's)	7 (89 g)	320	240
Eggrolls			
Beef steak teriyaki (Lo-An)	1 (78 g)	140	35
Chicken & Shrimp (Lo-An)	1 (78 g)	140	35
Chicken Munchers mini eggrolls (La Choy)	6 egg rolls (85g)	210	80
Egg roll bites (Matlaw's)	2 pieces (28g)	45	5
Lobster (Lo-An)	1 (78g)	150	35
Pork (Chung's)	2 (168g)	400	180
Shrimp Munchers mini eggrolls (La Choy)	6 egg rolls (85g)	190	60
Shrimp (Lo-An)	1 (78 g)	150	45
Vegetable (Barney's)	3 (81 g)	140	35
White meat – Chicken (Chung's)	2 (168 g)	340	100
White Meat chicken (Lo-An)	1 (78 g)	140	35
Potato Knishes	1 knish (210g)	436	150
Puffs			
Mushroom puffs (Mother's)	2 pieces (66g)	190	100
Potato puff (Manischewitz)	5 pieces (92g)	340	180
Spinach & potato puff (Manischewitz)	5 pieces (92g)	320	180
Spinach puffs (Mother's)	2 pieces (66g)	200	100
Quiche			
Petite quiche appetizers	6 (128 g)	370	190
Turnover			
Beef (Manischewitz)	4 pieces (85g)	300	190
BREADS			
New York Brand			
Texas Garlic toast with cheese	1 slice (40 g)	170	90
Pepperidge Farm			

Five cheese & garlic cheese bread	2 ¼" slices (56g)	200	90
Garlic toast	1 slice (40 g)	160	90
Mozzarella garlic cheese bread	2 ¼" slices (56g)	200	90
Sourdough garlic bread	2 ¼" slices (50g)	170	60
BREAKFAST FOODS			
Blintzes			
Empire kosher			
Apple	2 (124 g)	220	50
Cherry	2 (124 g)	200	35
Golden			
Blueberry	1 (62 g)	90	9
Cherry	1 (62 g)	95	9
Potato	1 (62 g)	90	36
Ratner's			
Blueberry cheese	1(61 g)	100	5
Cheese	1 (61 g)	90	5
Jumbo	1 (94.5 g)	133	6
Cherry	1 (61 g)	100	5
Potato	1 (61 g)	110	30
Breakfast burritos			
Bacon (Great starts, Swanson)	1 pkg (99g)	250	100
Breakfast sandwich			
Great starts (Swanson)			
Egg, Canadian bacon & cheese on a Muffin	1 pkg (116g)	290	140
French toast sticks with syrup	1 pkg (120g)	320	90
Pancake with bacon	1 pkg (128g)	400	180
Pancake with sausage	1 pkg (170g)	490	230
Sausage, egg & cheese on a biscuit	1 pkg (156g)	460	250
Scrambled eggs & bacon with Home-fried Potatoes	1 pkg (149g)	290	170
Scrambled eggs & sausage with Hashed brown Potatoes	1 pkg (177g)	360	230
Morningstar farms			
Breakfast links	2 links (45 g)	60	20
Breakfast patties	1 patty (38 g)	70	25
Breakfast strips	2 strips (16 g)	60	40
Grillers	1 patty (64 g)	140	60
Weight Watchers Smart ones			
English muffin sandwich	1 (113 g)	210	50
Handy Han & Cheese omelet	1 (113 g)	220	45
Croissants			
Original (Sara Lee)	1 (43 g)	170	70

French Toast, Frozen			
Aunt jemima, all types	2 (118 g)	240	60
Breakfast blast mini sticks (Swanson)	1 pkg (120g)	310	130
Downyflake			
Cinnamon Swirl	2 (113g)	270	50
Plain	2 (113g)	260	60
Great starts (Swanson)			
Cinnamon Swirl French Toast w/sausage	1 pkg (156g)	440	250
French Toast Sticks	1 pkg (120g)	320	90
French Toast w/sausage	1 pkg (156g)	410	230
DISHES OR DINNERS			
Amy's			
Burritos			
Cheese	1 burrito (170g)	280	5
Non-diary	1 burrito (170g)	250	70
California Veggie Burger	1 burger (72g)	100	25
Enchiladas			
Black bean, vegetable	1 enchilada (135g)	130	40
Cheese	1 enchilada (135g)	210	80
Spanish Rice & beans	1 meat (284 g)	250	70
Lasagna			
Tufu vegetable	1 lasagna (269 g)	300	90
Vegetable	1 lasagna (269 g)	300	90
Macaroni & cheese	1 entrée (255 g)	390	130
Mexican Tamale Pie	1 pie (227 g)	220	30
Pot Pies			
Beef	1 pie (198 g)	400	210
Broccoli	1 pie (213 g)	430	190
Vegetable	1 pie (213 g)	360	160
Shepherd's pie	1 pie (227 g)	160	35
Veggie Loaf	1 entrée (284 g)	260	50
Authentic Chinese Entrees			
Kung Pao Chicken	1 cup (199 g)	250	40
Moo Goo Gai Pan	1 cup (199 g)	260	70
Sweet & Sour Pork	1 cup (199 g)	250	40
Banquet			
Boneless Pork Riblet Meal	1 meal (283 g)	400	170
Brown Gravy& Salisbury Steaks	1 patty w/gravy (132 g)	230	150
Chicken Fried Beef Steak Meal	1 meal (283 g)	420	210
Chicken Nugget Meal	1 meal (191 g)	430	210

Chicken Pot Pie	1 pie (198 g)	380	200
Country Fried Chicken	3 oz (84 g)	270	160
Creamy Broccoli, Chicken & Cheese Meal	1 cup (219 g)	280	130
Fish Stick Meal	1 meal (187 g)	300	120
Fried Chicken	3 oz (84 g)	280	160
Fried Chicken Meal	1 meal (225 g)	470	240
Fried Chicken (the hearty one)	416 g	870	500
Grilled Chicken Meal	1 meal (280g)	330	120
Homestyle gravy & slicced turkey	2 slices w/gravy (134g)	120	70
Lasagna with meat sauce	1 cup (224 g)	350	100
Potato, ham, & broccoli au gratin	2/3 cup (140 g)	220	120
Salisbury steak meal	1 meal (269 g)	380	220
Salisbury steak meal (The hearty one)	1 meal (467 g)	780	490
Southern Fried Chicken	3 oz (84 g)	280	160
Turkey (mostly white meat) meal	1 meal (262 g)	280	90
Turkey (mostly white meat) meal (The hearty one)	1 meal (481 g)	630	290
Turkey pot pie	1 pie (198 g)	370	180
Birds Eye Easy Recipe			
Asian Stir Fry	2 ½ cups (253 g)		
	As packaged	230	15
	As prepared	330	90
Original Stir Fry	2 ¼ cups (270 g)		
	As packaged	210	35
	As prepared	300	100
Primavera	1 ¾ cups (215 g)		
	As packaged	180	45
	As prepared	250	80
Southwestern	1 ¾ cups (233 g)		
	As packaged	200	50
	As prepared	270	70
Teriyaki Stir Fry	2 cups (250 g)		
	As packaged	210	25
	As prepared	290	60
Birds Eye Pasta Secrets			
Italian Pesto	2 1/3 cups (181g) Frozen or 1 cup cooked	240	80
Primavera	2 1/3 cups (189g) Frozen or 1 cup cooked	230	90

Three cheese	2 cups (173 g) Frozen or 1 cup cooked	230	70
White cheddar	2 cups (180 g) Frozen or 1 cup cooked	240	90
Zesty Garlic	2 cups (167 g) Frozen or 1 cup cooked	240	90
Boca Burger (vegan)	1 burger (71 g)	84	0
Budget gourmet			
Beef pepper steak w/rice	1 entrée (255 g)	270	70
Cheese manicotti w/meat sauce	1 entrée (255 g)	350	170
Escalloped noodles & turkey	1 entrée (226 g)	320	150
Fettuccini Alfredo w/four cheese	1 entrée (226 g)	320	110
Italian sausage lasagna	1 entrée (283 g)	410	190
Macaroni & cheese (side dish)	1 pkg (163 g)	260	100
Rice pilaf w/green beans (side dish)	1 pkg (141 g)	220	90
Rigatoni in cream sauce w/broccoli & white chicken	1 entrée (226 g)	250	60
Roast beef supreme	1 entrée (255 g)	310	120
Spinach au gratin (side dish)	1 pkg (141 g)	160	110
Stir fry rice & vegetables	1 entrée (226g)	350	140
Spicy szechuan Vegetables & chicken	1 entrée (226 g)	290	80
Swedish meatballs	1 entrée (283 g)	550	310
Three cheese lasagna	1 entrée (255 g)	330	110
Budget Gourmet Low Fat			
Angel hair pasta	1 entrée (226 g)	230	45
Chicken oriental & vegetables	1 entrée (255 g)	290	70
Chinese style vegetable & chicken	1 entrée (226 g)	250	60
Fettuccini Primavera in Herb Sauce w/chicken	1 entrée (255 g)	280	70
Glazed turkey	1 entrée (255 g)	250	45
Italian style vegetables & chicken	1 entrée (226 g)	250	60
Linguini w/clams & shrimp	1 entrée (255 g)	280	70
Orange glazed chicken breast	1 entrée (255 g)	280	30
Pasta in wine & mushroom sauce w/chicken	1 entrée (255 g)	280	60
Penne pasta w/chunky tomatoes & Italian Sausage in sauce	1 entrée (226 g)	270	45
Rigatoni in cream sauce w/broccoli and White chicken	1 entrée (226 g)	250	60
Roast chicken w/herb gravy	1 meal (283 g)	260	70

Spaghetti narinara	1 entrée (226 g)	260	50
Ziti Parmesano	1 entrée (226 g)	260	60
Butterball Chicken Requests			
Italian style herb	1 piece (99 g)	190	60
Original	1 piece (99 g)	180	60
Parmesan	1 piece (99 g)	200	60
Celentano			
Broccoli stuffed shells	4 shells (280 g)	190	60
Cheese ravioli	6 ravioli (182 g)	360	35
Eggplant parmigiana	½ tray (196 g)	320	190
Eggplant rollettes	1 tray (280 g)	330	130
Low fat lasagna	1 tray (280 g)	260	25
Manicotti	1 pieces (196 g)	310	130
Stuffed shells	3 shells (196 g)	300	130
Dinty Moore			
Beef stew	1 cup (213 g)	190	90
Chicken and dumplings	1 cup (213 g)	200	50
Corned beef hash	1 cup (213 g)	350	200
Don Miguel			
Bean & cheese burrito	1 (198 g)	390	100
Bean & cheese chimichanga	1 (198 g)	470	160
Chicken & cheese burrito	1 (198 g)	410	130
Chicken burrito	1 (198 g)	360	70
Empire Kosher			
Breaded mushrooms	7 piece (81 g)	90	5
Breaded zucchini	7 pieces (83 g)	100	5
Chicken fat	1 tbsp (14 g)	120	120
Chicken pie	1 pie (227 g)	440	190
Chicken nuggets	5 nuggets (85 g)	180	80
Chicken stix	4 stix (88 g)	180	90
Ground turkey	4 oz (112 g)	150	70
Potato pancakes (Latkes)	1 piece (56 g)	100	40
Golden			
Potato pancakes (Latkes)	1 (38 g)	71	27
Gordon'			
Butterfly shrimp	20 (91 g)	240	120
Crunchy golden breaded fish fillets	1 fillet (108 g)	250	130
Crunchy golden fish sticks	6 sticks (104 g)	250	120

Garlic & herb breaded fish fillets	1 fillet (104 g)	220	100
Lemon pepper battered fish fillet	1 fillet (104 g)	270	160
Parmesan fish sticks	2 fillets (104 g)	260	140
Southern fried fish fillet	1 fillet (104 g)	230	130
Gordon's grilled fillets			
Italian herb	1 fillet (108mg)	130	50
All other flavors	1 fillet (108 g)	120	50
Gordon's Home style Baked Fillets			
Au gratin	1 fillet (131 g)	130	45
Garlic butter crumb	1 fillet (131 g)	170	80
Primavera	1 fillet (131 g)	120	45
Green Giant Create a Meal! Meal Starter			
Beefy noodle flavor	1 ¾ cups (178 g)		
	As packaged	170	15
	1 ¼ cups as prep.	350	130
Cheesy pasta & vegetable	1 ¾ cups (176 g)		
	As packaged	230	90
	1 ¼ cups as prep.	440	210
Country chicken noodle flavored with pasta	1 ¼ cups (176 g)		
	As packaged	130	5
Fajita style	1/3 packaged (168 g)	140	60
	2 fajitas as prep.	430	140
Hearty vegetable stew	1 ¼ cups (186 g)		
	As packaged	130	5
	1 ¼ cups as prep.	280	80
Homestyle Stew	1 ¼ cups (189 g)		
	As packaged	140	25
	Cup as prep.	340	140
Lo mein stir fry	2 1/3 cups (212 g)		
	As packaged	170	10
	1 ¼ cups as prep.	320	60
Oven roasted garlic herb	1 ¾ cups (184 g)		
	As packaged	160	0
	1 ¾ cups as prep.	360	80
Oven roasted homestyle pot roast	1 ¾ cups (191 g)		
	As packaged	150	5
	2 cups as prep.	370	120
Oven roasted savory onion	1 ¾ cups (185 g)		
	As packaged	130	10
	1 ¾ cups as prep.	340	120
Skillet lasagna	1 ¾ cups (188 g)		
	As packaged	160	5

	1 ¼ cups as prep.	350	120
Szechuan stir fry	1 ¾ cups (200 g)		
	As packaged	150	45
	1 ¼ cups as prep.	310	130
Teriyaki stir fry	1 ¾ cups (199 g)		
	As packaged	100	5
	1 ¼ cups as prep.	230	50
Green Giant Pasta Secrets			
Alfredo	2 cups (160 g) froz.		
	Or 1 cup cooked	260	90
Garlic seasoning	2 cups (188 g) froz.		
	Or 1 cup cooked	250	90
Lasagna style	2 cups (188 g) froz.		
	Or 1 cup cooked	260	90
White cheddar sauce	2 cups (18 g) froz.		
	Or 1 cup cooked	270	80
Healthy Choice			
Beef macaroni	1 meal (240 g)	220	35
Beef pepper steak oriental	1 meal (269 g)	250	35
Beef stroganoff	1 meal (311 g)	310	60
Beef tips, traditional	1 meal (318 g)	260	50
Breast of turkey, traditional	1 meal (298 g)	290	40
Cacciatore chicken	1 meal (354 g)	270	35
Charbroiled beef patty	1 meal (311 g)	280	50
Chicken & vegetables Marsala	1 meal (326 g)	240	35
Chicken breast con queso burrito	1 meal (299 g)	350	50
Chicken enchilada suprema	1 meal (320 g)	300	60
Chicken fettuccini alfredo	1 meal (240 g)	280	60
Chicken parmigiana	1 meal (326 g)	330	70
Chicken teriyaki	1 meal (311 g)	270	50
Country breaded chicken	1 meal (290 g)	350	80
Country glazed chicken	1 meal (240 g)	230	35
Country herb chicken	1 meal (344 g)	320	50
Country inn roast turkey	1 meal (283 g)	250	50
Country roast turkey w/mushrooms	1 meal (240 g)	220	35
Fiesta chicken fajitas	1 meal (198 g)	260	35
Ginger chicken hunan	1 meal (357 g)	380	45
Grilled chicken Sonoma	1 meal (255 g)	230	35
Grilled chicken w/mashed potatoes	1 meal (226 g)	170	30
Grilled glazed pork patty	1 meal (272 g)	300	60
Honey mustard chicken	1 meal (269 g)	270	35
Lemon pepper fish	1 meal (303 g)	320	60
Macaroni & cheese	1 meal (255 g)	320	60
Meatloaf, traditional	1 meal (340 g)	320	45
Mesquite chicken bbq	1 meal (298 g)	310	45

Pasta shells marinara	1 meal (340 g)	390	70
Penne pasta & roasted tomato sauce	1 meal (226 g)	230	45
Roasted chicken	1 meal (311 g)	230	45
Salisbury steak, traditional	1 meal (326 g)	330	60
Sesame chicken	1 meal (276 g)	240	25
Sesame chicken shanghai	1 meal (340 g)	300	45
Shrimp & vegetables maria	1 meal (354 g)	290	45
Southwestern grilled chicken	1 meal (289 g)	230	60
Spaghetti & sauce w/seasoned beef	1 meal (283 g)	280	50
Yankee pot roast	1 meal (311 g)	290	60
Zucchini lasagna	1 meal (383 g)	330	15
Hormel			
Beef stew	1 cup (213 g)	190	90
Chili, no beans	1 cup (209 g)	220	50
Macaroni & cheese	1 cup (213 g)	270	100
Noodles & chicken (Hearty Helpings)	1 cup (13 g)	250	140
Kid Cuisine			
Circus show corn dogs	1 meal (249 g)	450	140
Cosmic chicken nuggets	1 meal (257 g)	500	230
Game time taco roll-ups	1 meal (208 g)	420	160
High flying fried chicken	1 meal (286 g)	440	180
Magical macaroni & cheese	1 meal (300 g)	440	110
Pirate pizza w/cheese	1 meal (226 g)	430	100
Wave rider waffle sticks	1 meal (187 g)	380	70
Kids Fun Feast (Swanson)			
Chillin' cheese pizza	1 pkg (224 g)	350	80
Chompin' chicken drumlets	1 pkg (255 g)	490	220
Frazzlin' fried chicken	1 pkg (312 g)	660	320
Frenzied fish sticks	1 pkg (198 g)	370	130
Munchin' mini tacos	1 pkg (204 g)	390	140
Razzlin' rings	1 pkg (340 g)	390	100
Roarin' ravioli	1 pkg (312 g)	440	110
Kid's Kitchen (Hormel)			
Beans & wieners	1 cup (220 g)	310	110
Beefy mac	1 cup (213 g)	190	50
Kosherific			
Fish sticks	6 (113 g)	280	130
Lean Cuisine			
Baked chicken	1 pkg (244 g)	230	35

Baked fish	1 pkg (255 g)	270	50
Beef peppercornb	1 pkg (248 g)	220	60
Beef portabello	1 pkg (255 g)	220	60
Beef pot roast	1 pkg (255 g)	210	60
Cheese cannelloni	1 pkg (258 g)	230	35
Cheese lasagna with chicken breast scaloppini	1 pkg (283 g)	290	70
Cheese ravioli	1 pkg (240 g)	270	60
Chicken a l'orange	1 pkg (255 g)	250	15
Chicken & vegetables	1 pkg (297 g)	250	45
Chicken carbonara	1 pkg (255 g)	280	60
Chicken chow mein	1 pkg (255 g)	220	35
Chicken enchilada suiza	1 pkg (255 g)	280	40
Chicken fettuccine	1 pkg (262 g)	280	50
Chicken in wine sauce	1 pkg (230 g)	210	50
Chicken lasagna	1 pkg (283 g)	270	70
Chicken medallion with cheese sauce	1 pkg (265 g)	260	70
Chicken mediterranean	1 pkg (265 g)	260	70
Chicken parmesan	1 pkg (308 g)	220	40
Chicken in peanut sauce	1 pkg (255 g)	290	50
Chicken piccata	1 pkg (255 g)	270	60
Chicken pie	1 pkg (269 g)	290	80
Chicken with basil cream sauce	1 pkg (240 g)	270	60
Classic cheese lasagna	1 pkg (326 g)	270	35
Fettuccini Alfredo	1 pkg (262 g)	300	60
Glazed chicken	1 pkg (240 g)	240	50
Glazed turkey tenderloins	1 pkg (255 g)	240	40
Grilled chicken & penne pasta	1 pkg (265 g)	260	70
Grilled chicken salsa	1 pkg (251 g)	270	60
Herb roasted chicken	1 pkg (226 g)	210	40
Home style turkey	1 pkg (265 g)	230	40
Honey roasted chicken	1 pkg (240 g)	290	50
Honey roasted pork	1 pkg (269 g)	250	50
Lasagna with meat sauce	1 pkg (297 g)	290	60
Macaroni and cheese	1 pkg (283 g)	290	60
Meatloaf	1 pkg (265 g)	250	60
Oriental-style dumplings	1 pkg (255 g)	300	50
Oven roasted beef	1 pkg (262 g)	260	70
Roasted turkey breast	1 pkg (276 g)	270	20
Salisbury steak	1 pkg (269 g	280	70
Southern beef tips	1 pkg (248 g)	290	50
Spaghetti with meat sauce	1 pkg (326 g)	290	45
Shrimp & angel hair pasta	1 pkg (283 g)	290	50
Swedish meatballs	1 pkg (258 g)	290	50
Three-bean chili	1 pkg (283 g)	250	50

Vegetable eggroll	1 pkg (255 g)	340	60
Lean Cuisine Great for Lunch			
Alfredo pasta primavera	1 pkg (283 g)	290	60
Broccoli & cheddar cheese sauce			
Over baked potato	1 pkg (290 g)	250	80
Cheese lasagna casserole	1 pkg (283 g)	270	50
Mandarin chicken	1 pkg (255 g)	250	35
Penne pasta with tomato basil sauce	1 pkg (283 g)	70	30
Roasted potatoes with broccoli and cheddar			
Cheese sauce	1 pkg (290 g	260	50
Teriyaki stir-fry	1 pkg (283 g)	290	30
Lean Cuisine Hearty Portions			
Cheese & spinach manicotti	1 pkg (439 g)	340	60
Chicken & barbecue sauce	1 pkg (393 g)	380	50
Chicken Florentine	1 pkg (395 g)	420	80
Grilled beef patty & gravy with			
Whipped poitatioes	1 pkg (439 g)	370	80
Grilled chicken & penne pasta	1 pkg (396 g)	380	60
Lasagna	1 pkg (425 g)	440	80
Roasted chicken with mushrooms	1 pkg (354 g)	380	60
Roasted turkey breast	1 pkg (396 g)	290	45
Mama Lucias			
Italian style meatballs	3 (84 g)	270	190
Marie Cdallender's			
Beef tips in mushroom sauce	1 meal (385 g)	430	170
Breaded chicken parmigiana dinner	1 dinner (454 g)	620	250
Chicken (white meat) & broccoli pot pie	1 cup (290 g)	710	440
Chicken cordon bleu	1 meal (368 g)	590	230
Chicken pot pie	1 cup (241 g)	520	290
Chili & cornbread	1 cup + 1.5 oz		
	Cornbread (297g)	350	120
Chunky chicken & noodle	1 meal (368 g)	520	270
Country fried chicken & gravy	1 meal (454 g)	620	270
Fettuccini primavera with tortellini	1 cup (234 g)	430	240
Fetrruccini with broccoli & chickenb in			
Alfredo sauce	1 cup (221 g)	410	220
Grilled chicken in mushrool sauce	1 dinner (397 g)	480	140
Grilled turkey breast strips & rice pilaf	1 meal (333 g)	310	90
Herb roasted chicken	1 dinner (397 g)	670	380
Lasagna with meat sauce	1 cup (246 g)	370	170
Macaroni & cheese	1 meal (382 g)	510	160
Meatloaf & gravy	1 meal (397 g)	540	270
with mashed potatoes			
Sirloin Salisbury steak & gravy	1 meal (397 g)	550	220
Spaghetti & meat sauce	1 cup + 2 oz garlic		

	Bread (290 g)	380	120
Stuffed pasta trio	1 meal (297 g)	380	160
Swedish meatballs	1 meal (354 g)	520	240
Turkey pot pie	1 cup (280 g)	600	320
Turkey with gravy & dressing	1 meal (397 g)	500	170
Matlaw's			
Stuffed clams	1 clam (71 g)	120	50
Michelina"s			
Chicken Italiano with Parmesan cheese	1 pkg (213 g)	250	60
Chili Mac	1 container (227g)	270	80
Gravy with egg noodles and Swedish meatballs	1 pkg (284 g)	360	110
Fettuccine alfredo	1 pkg (269 g)	410	150
Four cheese lasagna	1 pkg (277 g)	290	70
Lasagna with meat sauce	1 pkg (255 g)	300	70
Linguini with clams	1 pkg (255 g)	310	30
Macaroni & beef	1 container (227g)	250	60
Macaroni & cheese	1 container (227g)	340	120
Penne pollo	1 pkg (255 g)	320	80
Pepper steak & rice	1 pkg (241 g)	270	40
Rigatoni pomodoro	1 container (227g)	220	20
Salisbury steak & gravy	1 pkg (241 g)	300	160
Spaghetti Bolognese	1 pkg (255 g)	290	35
Wheels & cheese	1 container (227g)	300	80
Michelina's Lean'n tasty			
Black bean chili	1 pkg (284 g)	400	45
Fettuccine with creamy pesto sauce	1 pkg (241 g)	250	60
Glazed chicken	1 pkg (227 g)	280	30
Gravy with egg noodles & Swedish Meatballs	1 pkg (284 g)	300	60
Honey barbecue sauce with chicken & rice	1 pkg (241 g)	300	20
Mac & beef	1 pkg (227 g)	230	50
Macaroni & cheese	1 pkg (227 g)	270	60
Penne arrabiata	1 pkg (255 g)	230	20
Penne pasta with mushrooms	1 pkg (227 g)	250	50
Spaghetti & meatballs with tomato sauce	1 pkg (255 g)	290	60
Spaghetti with onions, green peppers & mushrooms	1 pkg (255 g)	280	50
Teriyaki chicken with rice	1 pkg (241 g)	290	25
Mrs. Budd's			
Chicken a la king	1 cup (238 g)	420	80

Chicken supreme	1 cup (238 g)	430	100
White meat chicken pie fancy vegetables	1 cup (227 g)	310	140
Original recipe	1 cup (227 g)	330	150
Mrs. Paul's			
Devil crabs	1 cake (82 g)	170	60
Egg plant parmigiana	½ cup (118 g)	190	100
Grilled salmon creamy dill	1 fillet (92 g)	90	25
Honey mustard	1 fillet (92 g)	90	15
Grilled tuna			
Barbecue	1 fillet (92 g)	100	5
Sesame teriyaki	1 fillet (92 g)	110	15
Mrs. Paul's Dream Kitchen			
Crispy crunchy fish fillets	2 fillets (106 g)	240	110
Crispy crunch fish sticks	6 sticks (95 g)	210	90
Mrs. Paul's Grilled Fillets			
Garlic butter	1 fillet (104 g)	130	50
Lemon pepper	1 fillet (104 g)	130	50
Mrs. Paul's Premium Fillets			
Flounder	1 fillet (80 g)	170	70
Haddock	1 fillet (120 g)	230	100
Nancy's Quiche			
Quiche Florentine	1 quiche (170 g)	440	230
Quiche lorraine	1 quiche (170 g)	470	240
Petite Quiche appetizers all types	6 (128 g)	370	200
Natural Touch			
Garden veggie patty	1 patty (67 g)	100	25
Patio Burritos			
Bean & cheese	1 burrito (142 g)	300	80
Beef & bean	1 burrito (142 g)	320	110
Chicken	1 burrito (142 g)	290	70
Patio Diners			
Cheese enchilada dinner	1 meal (340 g)	370	110
Fiesta dinner	1 meal (340 g)	350	100
Mexican style dinner	1 meal (376 g)	470	170
Quiche St. Jacques			
Quiche jardinière	1/11 of 9" diameter		

	Quiche (57 g)	160	100
Quiche lorraine	1/11 of 9" diameter		
	Quiche (57 g)	170	110
Quiche maximillian	1/11of 9" diameter		
	Quiche (57 g)	160	110
Quiche provencal	1/11 of 9" diameter		
	Quiche (57 g)	160	100
Safeway Select Gourmet Club			
St. Louis style pork spareribs	2 ribs (125 g)	370	210
Veal cannelloni	1 piece (189 g)	250	100
Sea Pak			
Clam strips	1 pkg (141 g)	410	200
Jumbo butterfly shrimp	4 shrimp (85 g)	200	80
Popcorn shrimp	15 shrimp (85 g)	210	110
Spare the Rib			
Pork, no bones	5 oz (140 g)	380	260
Stouffer's			
Baked chicken breast (home style)	1 pkg (251 g)	260	100
Breaded pork cutlet (home style)	1 pkg (283 g)	420	200
Cheddar pasta with beef & tomatoes	1 pkg (311 g)	500	210
Cheese ravioli	1 pkg (301 g)	380	120
Chicken a la king	1 pkg (269 g)	350	110
Chicken & dumplings (home style)	1 pkg (283 g)	280	70
Chicken breast in barbecue sauce (home style)	1 pkg (283 g)	510	210
Chicken breast with mushroom gravy	1 pkg (283 g)	360	130
Chicken parmigiana (home style)	1 pkg (340 g)	460	140
Chicken pie	1 pkg (283 g)	540	290
	1 cup (250 g)	500	280
Chili with beans	1 pkg (248 g)	290	90
Chunky beef & tomatoes (home style)	1 pkg (283 g)	280	80
Country style biscuit	1 pkg (255 g)	510	260
Creamed chip beef	½ cup (125 g)	160	100
Escalloped apples	2/3 cup (158 g)	190	25
Escalloped chicken and noodles	1 pkg (283 g)	430	240
Fettuccini alfredo	1 pkg (283 g)	520	250
Fish fillet (home style)	1 pkg (255 g)	430	190
Five cheese lasagna	1 pkg (304 g)	360	120
Fried chicken breast (home style)	1 pkg (251 g)	400	150
Green pepper steak	1 pkg (297 g)	320	80
Lasagna bake with meat sauce	1 cup (290 g)	370	100
Lasagna with meat & sauce	1 cup (215 g)	260	90
Lasagna with tomato sauce &	1 pkg (308 g)	340	100

Italian Sausage			
Macaroni and beef	1 pkg (326 g)	340	80
Macaroni and cheese	1 cup (225 g)	320	140
Macaroni and cheese with broccoli	1 pkg (297 g)	360	150
Meatloaf (home style)	1 pkg (279 g)	390	180
Roast turkey breast (home style)	1 pkg (272 g)	310	110
Salisbury steak (home style)	1 pkg (272 g)	380	160
Sliced beef brisket (home style)	1 pkg (283 g)	370	150
Spaghetti with meatballs	1 pkg (357 g)	440	130
Spaghetti with meat sauce	1 pkg (272 g)	350	100
Stuffed peppers	1 pepper & sauce (220 g)	180	70
Swedish meatballs with pasta	1 pkg (290 g)	480	210
Tuna noodle casserole	1 pkg (283 g)	340	130
Turkey tetrazzini	1 pkg (283 g)	360	150
Veal parmigiana (Home style)	1 pkg (329 g)	430	150
Vegetable lasagna	1 pkg (297 g)	440	180
Welsh rarebit	¼ cup (62 g)	120	80
Stouffer's Family Style Favorites			
Lasagna with meat sauce	1 cup (215 g)	270	80
Macaroni & cheese	1 cup (255 g)	380	150
Stouffer's Hearty Portions			
Beef pot roast	1 pkg (453 g)	430	160
Country fried beef steak	1 pkg (453 g)	750	370
Pork with roast potatoes	1 pkg (453 g)	570	140
Roast beef	1 pkg (453 g)	430	160
Salisbury steak	1 pkg (453 g)	630	260
Sliced turkey breast	1 pkg (453 g)	570	240
Swanson Classic Mac and More			
Macaroni & cheese	1 pkg (170 g)	240	80
Swanson Dinners			
Beef pot pie	1 pkg (198 g)	415	210
Boneless pork rib	1 pkg (298 g)	470	170
Chicken nuggets	1 pkg (284 g)	590	230
Chicken pot pie	1 pie (198 g)	410	200
Country fried beef steak	1 pkg (305 g)	460	200
Fish 'n chips	1 pkg (284 g)	490	180
Fried chicken			
Dark portions	1 pkg (312 g)	580	270
White portions	1 pkg (312 g)	630	280
Meatloaf	1 pkg (305 g)	380	130

Salisbury steak	1 pkg (312 g)	340	140
Sirloin beef tips	1 pkg (47 g)	450	140
Turkey (mostly white meat)	1 pkg (333 g)	320	70
Turkey pot pie	1 pie (198 g)	400	190
Veal parmigiana	1 pkg 319 g)	390	160
Yankee pot toast	1 pkg (326 g)	250	40
Swanson Hungry man			
Beef pot pie	1 pkg (397 g)	660	299
Boneless chicken	1 pkg (489 g)	630	200
Boneless pork rib	1 pkg (400 g)	770	340
Chicken pot pie	1 pkg (397 g)	650	320
Country fried beef steak	1 pkg (454 g)	660	300
Fisherman's platter	1 pkg (368 g)	650	230
Fried chicken (mostly white meat)	1 pkg (439 g)	800	350
Salisbury steak	1 pkg (454 g)	360	50
Turkey (mostly white meat)	1 pkg (475 g)	10	130
Turkey pot pie	1 pkg (397 g)	650	310
Taj Gourmet			
Bean masala	1 pkg (342 g)	330	50
Chicken korma	1 pkg (312 g)	330	80
Chicken tikka masala	1 pkg (312 g)	330	80
Dal bahaar	1 pkg (342 g)	330	60
Palak paneer	1 pkg (342 g)	320	60
Vegetable korma	1 pkg (342 g)	320	50
Tyson			
Beef fajitas	3 ½ fajitas (357 g)	480	120
Van De Kamp's			
Baked breaded fish fillets	2 fillets (99 g)	150	25
Battered fish fillets	1 fillet (75 g)	180	100
Breaded fish fillets	2 fillets (99 g)	280	170
Breaded fish sticks	6 sticks (114 g)	290	150
Garlic & herb baked breaded fish fillets	1 fillet (78 g)	150	45
Lemon pepper baked breaded fish fillets	1 fillet (78 g)	140	45
Weight Watchers Smart Ones			
Angel hair pasta	1 entrée (225 g)	180	20
Bowtie pasta & mushrooms marsala	1 entrée (273 g)	270	60
Broccoli and cheese baked potato	1 entrée (283 g)	250	50
Chicken Fettuccini	1 entrée (283 g)	300	60
Creamy Rigatoni with broccoli & chicken	1 entrée (255 g)	230	20
Fiesta chicken	1 entrée (241 g)	210	20
Grilled Salisbury steak	1 entrée (241 g)	250	80

Home style macaroni & cheese	1 entrée (255 g)	280	60
Hunan style rice & vegetables	1 entrée (293 g)	280	70
Lasagna Florentine	1 entrée (283 g)	200	20
Lemon herb chicken piccata	1 entrée (241 g)	200	20
Macaroni and cheese	1 entrée (255 g)	220	20
Pasta & spinach romano	1 entrée (293 g)	260	70
Pasta with tomato basil sauce	1 entrée (272 g)	260	60
Penne pasta with sundried tomatoes	1 entrée (282 g)	280	70
Penne pollo	1 entrée (283 g)	290	50
Ravioli Florentine	1 entrée (241 g)	220	20
Roast turkey medallions	1 entrée (241 g)	180	20
Santa fe style rice & beans	1 entrée (283 g)	290	70
Shrimp marinara	1 entrée (255 g)	180	20
Swedish meatballs	1 entrée (255 g)	300	90
Tuna noodle casserole	1 entrée (269 g)	270	60
Yu Sing (Michelina's)			
Chicken fried rice	1 pkg (227 g)	360	70
Chicken lo mein	1 meal (227 g)	230	40
Oriental beef & peppers	1 pkg (227 g)	290	60
Shrimp fried rice	1 pkg (227 g)	360	50
Shrimp lo mein	1 pkg (227 g)	220	15
Sweet & sour chicken	1 pkg (241 g)	340	35
PIZZAS, FROZEN			
Amy's Pizza			
Cheese	1/3 pizza (123 g)	310	100
Spinach	1/3 pizza (132 g)	320	100
Vegetable, no cheese	1/3 pizza (113 g)	270	70
Celeste Pizza-for-One			
Cheese	1 pizza (170 g)	420	180
Deluxe	1 pizza (202 g)	470	220
Four cheese			
Original	1 pizza (174 g)	480	240
Zesty	1 pizza (174 g)	470	210
Pepperoni	1 pizza (170 g)	470	240
Suprema	1 pizza (221 g)	530	260
Vegetable	1 pizza (187 g)	420	180
Di Giorno			
Four cheese			
Small	1/3 pizza (114 g)	280	90
Large	1/6 pizza (139 g)	330	100
Pepperoni			

Small	1/3 pizza (120 g)	320	120
Large	1/6 pizza (148 g)	390	150
Spinach, mushroom & garlic	1/3 pizza (125 g)	270	80
Supreme	1/6 pizza (165 g)	400	150
Fox De Luxe			
Sausage & Pepperoni	1 pizza (184 g)	460	160
Healthy Choice French Bread Pizza			
Cheese	1 pizza (170 g)	340	45
Pepperoni	1 pizza (170 g)	340	45
Supreme	1 pizza (180 g)	330	45
Vegetable	1 pizza (170 g)	280	35
Hot Pockets			
Pizza Mini's			
Double cheese	6 pieces (85 g)	240	80
Pepperoni	6 pieces (85 g)	250	100
Sausage & pepperoni	6 pieces (85 g)	230	80
Pizza snacks			
Pepperoni	6 pieces (85 g)	220	70
Toaster Breaks Pizza			
Double cheese	1 piece (60 g)	190	80
Pepperoni	1 piece (60 g)	200	90
Jeno's Crisp 'n Tasty Pizza			
Chompin' cheese	1 pizza (195 g)	460	170
Crazy combination (sausage & Pepperoni)	1 pizza (198 g)	520	250
Power pepperoni	1 pizza (192 g)	510	240
Lean Cuisine French Bread Pizza			
Deluxe	1 pkg (183 g)	300	50
Pepperoni	1 pkg (148 g)	310	60
Mama Celeste			
Four cheese	1/6 pizza (140 g)	340	90
Pepperoni	1/6 pizza (142 g)	380	140
Supreme	1/6 pizza (157 g)	380	150
McCain Ellio's			
Cheese	1 slice (75 g)	160	45
Ore Ida Bagel Bites			
Cheese & pepperoni	4 pieces (88 g)	200	60
Cheese, sausage & pepperoni	4 pieces (88 g)	190	60
Three cheese	4 pieces (88 g)	190	50

Red Baron Deep Dish Singles Pizzas			
Cheese	1 pizza (168 g)	500	230
Pepperoni	1 pizza (168 g)	540	280
Supreme	1 pizza (168 g)	490	240
Safeway Select Gourmet Club			
French bread pepperoni pizza	1 pizza (85 g)	230	90
Stouffer's French Bread Pizza			
Cheese	1 pizza (147 g)	370	150
Deluxe	1 pizza (175 g)	420	160
Extra cheese	1 pizza (167 g)	400	140
Five cheese	1 pizza (147 g)	370	150
Grilled vegetable	1 pizza (165 g)	350	100
Pepperoni	1 pizza (159 g)	390	140
Pepperoni & mushroom	1 pizza (174 g)	440	170
Sausage & pepperoni	1 pizza (177 g)	470	200
Three meat (sausage, pepperoni, bacon)	1 pizza (177 g)	470	200
Tombstone			
Light			
Vegetable	1/5 pizza (131 g)	240	60
Original			
Pepperoni	¼ pizza (152 g)	400	190
Supreme	1/5 pizza (130 g)	320	140
Thin crust			
Four meat combination	¼ pizza (143 g)	380	200
Pepperoni	¼ pizza (138 g)	400	230
Tombstone for One Deep Dish Pizza			
Cheese	1 pizza (177 g)	470	190
Pepperoni	1 pizza (177 g)	510	240
Chef America (cont.)			
Pepperoni & Sausage Pizza	1 piece (128 g)	330	120
Pepperoni Pizza	1 piece (1 28 g)	360	140
Tyson (cont.)			
Breaded Chicken Breast Tenders	3 tenders (92 g)	100	0
Chicken Faiitas	3 ½ fajitas (374 g)	460	100
Hot 'n Spicy Chicken Wings	4 pcs (96 g)	220	130
Mandarin Sesame Wraps	½ wraps (416 g)	630	140
Wamplers			
100% Pure Ground Chicken	4 oz (112 g)	220	120
100% Pure Ground Turkey	4 oz (112 g)	210	130
100% Pure Turkey Burgers	1 burger (112 g)	210	130

Turkey Mignons	1 mignon (142 g)	230	110
SANDWICHES			
Amy's In a Pocket Sandwich			
Spinach Feta	1 (1 28 g)	200	60
Vegetable Pie	1 (1 42 g)	230	60
Banquet Hot Sandwich Toppers			
Creamed Chipped Beef	1 bag (113 g)	120	50
Gravy & Salisbury Steak	1 bag (141 g)	210	40
Gravy & Sliced Beef	1 bag (113 g)	70	0
Gravy & Sliced Turkey	1 bag (141 g)	160	00
Bob Evans Farms			
Sausage & Biscuit	2 sandwiches (112 g)	370	210
Chef America			
Croissant Pockets			
Chicken, Broccoli & Cheddar	1 piece (128 g)	290	80
Egg, Sausage & Cheese	1 piece (128 g)	340	130
Ham & Cheese	1 piece (128 g)	320	110
Pepperoni Pizza	1 piece (128 g)	360	140
Turkey & Ham with Swiss	1 piece (128 g)	290	90
Hot Pockets			
Beef & Cheddar	1 piece (128 g)	350	150
Beef with Barbecue	1 piece (128 g)	340	110
Chicken & Cheddar with Broccoli	1 piece (128 g)	300	90
Meatballs with Mozzarella	1 piece (128 g)	320	100
Lean Pockets			
Chicken Broccoli Supreme	1 piece (128 g)	260	60
Chicken Fajita	1 piece (128 g)	270	60
Chicken Parmesan	1 piece (128 g)	280	60
Ham & Cheddar	1 piece (128 g)	280	70
Pepperoni Pizza Deluxe (reduced fat)	1 piece (128 g)	270	60
Philly Steak & Cheese	1 piece (128 g)	260	60
Turkey, Broccoli & Cheese	1 piece (1 28 g)	250	60
Toaster Breaks Melts			
Ham & Cheese	1 piece (61 g)	180	80
Veggie Pockets			
Bar-B-Q Style	1 pocket (127g)	290	50
Broccoli & Cheddar Style	1 pocket (127 g)	290	80
Greek Style	1 pocket (127 g)	250	80
Indian Style	1 pocket (127 g)	260	80

Oriental Style	1 pocket (127 g)	250	80
Pizza Style	1 pocket (127 g)	270	50
Tex-Mex Style	1 pocket (127 g)	280	80
Veggie Burger	1 sandwich (71 g)	130	10
Gardenburger Veggie Patties			
Fire Roasted Vegetable	1 patty (71 g)	120	25
Gardenburger with Cheese	1 patty (71 g)	110	25
Savory Mushroom	1 patty (71 g)	120	25
The Original	1 patty (71 g)	130	25
Veggie Medley	1 patty (71 g)	100	0
Green Giant Harvest Burgers			
Original flavor	1 patty (90 g)	140	35
Healthy Choice Hearty Handfuls			
Chicken & Broccoli	1 hearty handful (173 g)	320	50
Chicken & Mushrooms	1 hearty handful (173 g)	310	45
Garlic Chicken	1 hearty handful (173 g)	330	45
Ham & Cheese	1 hearty handful (173 g)	320	45
Italian Style Meatball	1 hearty handful (173 g)	320	45
Philly Beef Steak	1 hearty handful (173 g)	290	45
Jimmie Dean			
Bacon, Egg, & Cheese on a Biscuit	1 sandwich (102 g)	300	150
Sausage, Egg, & Cheese on a Biscuit	1 sandwich (128 g)	390	240
Sausage Biscuits	2 sandwiches (113 g)	390	220
Morningstar Farms			
Better 'n Burgers	1 patty (78 g)	70	0
Chik Nuggets	4 nuggets (86 g)	160	40
Chik Patties	1 patty (71 g)	150	50
Garden Veggie Patties	1 patty (67 g)	100	25
Spicy Black Bean	1 patty (78 g)	110	10
Veggle Dogs	1 link (57 g)	80	5
Quaker Maid			
Italian Meatball Sandwich	1 (170 g)	460	220
Philly Cheese Steak	1 sandwich (170 g)	400	80
Pure Beef Sandwich Steak	1 steak (56 g)	170	130

Safeway Stuffed Sandwiches			
Barbecue Beef	1 piece (127 g)	310	120
Ham & Cheese	1 piece (128 g)	320	140
Lean Turkey, Broccoli & Cheddar	1 piece (128 g)	240	60
Pepperoni Pizza	1 piece (128 g)	370	170
Steak-umm			
100% All Beef Sandwich Steaks	1 steak, raw (57 g)	190	150
Reduced Fat Real Beef Sandwich Steaks	1 steak, raw (57 g)	110	63
Green Giant (cont.)			
Rice Pilaf	1 pkg (283 g)	260	25
Shoepeg White Corn & Butter	¼ cup (112 g)	120	25
Southwestern Style Corn & Roasted Red Peppers	¼ cup (99 g)	90	10
Teriyaki Vegetables	¼ cup (110 g)	100	60
Vegetable Medley & Butter	¼ cup (103 g)	60	20
White & Wild Rice	1 pkg (283 g)	280	50
Ore Ida			
Country Style Hash Browns	¼ cup (91 g)	80	0
Country Style Potato Wedges	13 pieces (84 g)	120	40
Country Style Steak Fries	8 pieces (84 g)	110	30
Crispers	17 fries (84 g)	220	110
Golden Crinkles	14 pieces (84 g)	120	30
Golden Fries	16 pieces (84 g)	120	35
Golden Patties Shredded Potatoes	1 patty (71 g)	140	70
Mashed Potatoes	¼ cup (69 g)	90	20
Mini Tater Tots	19 pieces (84 g)	180	90
Onion Ringers	6 rings (88 g)	210	100
Onion Rings	4 pieces (84 g)	220	100
Oven Chips	7 pieces (84 g)	180	70
Potato Wedges with skins	pieces (84 g)	110	25
Shoestrings	44 pieces (84 g)	150	50
Tater Tots	9 pieces (86 g)	150	60
Toaster Hash Browns	2 patties (99 g)	190	90
Topped Baked Potatoes, Broccoli & Cheese	½ baker (159 g)	160	35
Twice Baked Potatoes Cheddar cheese	1 piece (141 g)	190	70
Sour cream & chives	1 piece (I 41 g)	190	60
Safeway Select Side Dish			
BBQ Beans	½ cup	200	15
Cheddar Cheese & Bacon			

Mashed Potatoes	½ cup	190	90
AU BON PAIN			
Breads			
Bagels			
Cinnamon Raisin	1	280	9
Plain, Onion, or Sesame	1	270	9
Loaf			
Baguette	1 loaf	810	18
Cheese	1 loaf	1670	261
Four Grain	1 loaf	1420	99
Onion Herb	1 loaf	1430	117
Parisienne	1 loaf	1490	36
Muffins			
Blueberry	1	390	99
Bran	1	390	99
Carrot	1	450	198
Corn	1	460	153
Cranberry Walnut	1	350	117
Oat Bran Apple	1	400	90
Pumpkin	1	410	144
Whole Grain	1	440	144
Rolls			
Alpine	1	220	27
Country Seed	1	220	36
Hearth	1	250	18
Petit Pain	1	220	9
Pumpernickel	1	210	18
Rye	1	230	18
3 Seed Raisin	1	250	36
Vegetable	1	230	45
Sandwich			
Braided Roll	1 roll	387	99
Croissant	1 roll	300	126
French Sandwich	1 roll	320	9
Hearth Sandwich	1 roll	370	27
Multigrain Slice	2 slices	391	27
Pita Pocket	1 pocket	80	9
Rye Slice	2 slices	374	36

Cookies			
Chocolate Chip	1 serving	280	135
Chocolate Chunk Pecan	1 serving	290	153
Oatmeal Raisin	1 serving	250	81
Peanut Butter	1 serving	290	135
White Chocolate Chunk Pecan	1 serving	300	153
Croissants			
Dessert			
Almond	1	420	225
Apple	1	250	90
Blueberry Cheese	1	380	180
Chocolate	1	400	216
Cinnamon Raisin	1	390	117
Coconut Pecan	1	440	207
Hazelnut Chocolate	1	480	252
Plain	1	220	90
Strawberry or Raspberry Cheese	1	400	180
Sweet Cheese	1	420	207
Hot Filled			
Ham & Cheese	1	370	180
Spinach & Cheese	1	290	144
Turkey & Cheddar	1	410	198
Turkey & Havarti	1	410	189
Salads			
Chicken Tarragon Garden	1	310	135
Cracked Pepper Chicken Garden	1	100	18
Grilled Chicken Garden	1	110	18
Large Garden	1	40	9
Shrimp Garden	1	102	18
Small Garden	1	20	9
Tuna Garden	1	350	225
Salad Dressings			
Balsamic Vinaigrette	2.25 oz	311	297
Champagne Vinegrette	2.25 oz	251	234
County Blue Cheese	2.25 oz	325	279
Honey with Poppy Seed	2.25 oz	351	315
Low Cal Italian	2.25 oz	68	54
Olive Oil Caesar	2.25 oz	255	144
Parmesan & Pepper	2.25 oz	235	189
Sesame French	2.25 oz	339	243
Tomato Basil	2.25 oz	66	9

Sandwich Fillings

Cheese			
Brie Cheese	1 serving	300	216
Dark meat chicken			
Without skin	95 g	190	90
With skin	125 g	320	190
½ chicken with skin	277 g	590	300
Baked Italian pasta	¼ cup (170 g)	190	80
BBQ baked beans	¼ cup (201 g)	270	45
Brownie	1 piece (95 g)	450	240
Butternut squash	¼ cup (193 g)	160	60
Caesar salad			
Entree	1 (283 g)	510	380
Without dressing	1 (225 g)	230	110
Side	1 (113 g)	200	159
Chicken Caesar salad	1 (369 g)	650	410
Chicken gravy	28 g	15	10
Chicken noodle soup	1 cup (257 g)	130	40
Chicken potpie	1 pie (425 g)	780	410
Chicken salad sandwich	1 (327 g)	680	270
Chicken sandwich			
With cheese & sauce	1 (352 g)	750	300
Without cheese & sauce	1 (281 g)	430	40
Chicken tortilla soup	1 cup (238 g)	220	100
Chocolate chip cookie	1 (79 g)	340	150
Chunky chicken salad	¼ cup (58 g)	370	240
Cinnamon apple pie	1s pie (1 36 g)	390	200
Corn bread	1 loaf (68 g)	200	50
Creamed spinach	¼ cup (181 g)	260	180
Fruit salad	¼ cup (156 g)	70	5
Green bean casserole	¼ cup (170 g)	130	80
Ham & turkey club			
With cheese & sauce	1 (379 g)	890	390
Without cheese & sauce	1 (266 g)	420	50
Ham sandwich			
With cheese & sauce	1 (337 g)	750	310
Without cheese & sauce	1 (266 g)	440	70
Hearth honey ham	142 g	210	80
Homestyle mashed potatoes	2/3 cup (161 g)	190	80
with gravy	3/4 cup (1 89 g)	210	90

CHAIN FAMILY-STYLE RESTAURANTS, such as Applebee's, Bennigans, Chili's, TGI Friday's, Grady's American Grill, Hard Rock Cafe, Houlihan's, Houston's, and Ruby Tuesday*

Appetizers			
Buffalo Wings	12 wings	700	432
Chili	½ cup	350	144
Fried Mozzarella Sticks	9 sticks	830	459
Stuffed Potato Skins	8 skins	1120	711
Entrees			
Beef			
BBQ Baby Back Ribs	14 ribs	1120	711
Hamburger	1	770	486
Mushroom Cheeseburger	1	660	324
Sirloin Steak	7 oz	900	513
Steak Fajitas with Tortillas	1 order 410	180	
With guacamote, sour cream, & cheese			
Chicken			
Bacon & Cheese Grilled Chicken Sandwich	1	650	270
Chicken Caesar Salad with dressing	4 cups	660	414
Chicken Fajitas with Tortillas	1 order	840	216
With guacamote, sour cream, & cheese		1170	504
Chicken Fingers	5 pieces	620	306
Grilled Chicken	6 oz	270	72
With loaded baked potato & vegetables		950	378
Oriental Chicken Salad with dressing	4 cups	750	441
Side Orders			
Cole Slaw	1 cup	170	126
French Fries	2 cups	590	279
Loaded Baked Potato	1	620	279
Onion Rings	11	900	576
Vegetable of the Day	1 cup	60	27
Dessert			
Fudge Brownie Sundae	10 oz	1130	513
CHILI'S			
Chicken fajitas	1 order	870	306

Chicken sandwich	1	1082	450
Diet by Chocolate cake with hot fudge sauce	1 slice	370	15
Grilled chicken platter	1	757	189
Guiltless Grill			
Chicken fajitas	1 order	690	54
Chicken platter	1	450	32
Chicken salad	1	254	30
Chicken sandwich	1	485	47
Tuna sandwich	1	950	342
CHINESE RESTAURANT			
Barbecued pork (not fried)	1 whole dish	1374	986
Beef with vegetables	1 whole dish	1863	1232
Chicken with cashews	1 whole dish	1572	1068
Chicken with vegetables	1 whole dish	1765	1075
Chinese Noodle Soup	1 whole dish	1224	652
Egg rolls	serving	265	81
Hot and sour soup		152	103
Hunan shrimp (not fried)	serving	165	72

BEVERAGES

Coffee Drinks

Caffe Latte			
Short			
with whole milk	8 fl oz	140	60
with lowfat milk	8 fl oz	110	35
with nonfat milk	8 ft oz	80	0
with soy milk	8 fl oz	70	35
Tall			
with whole milk	12 fl oz	210	100
with lowfat milk	12 fl oz	170	50
with nonfat milk	12 fl oz	120	0
with soy milk	12 fl oz	110	60
Grande			
with whole milk	16 fl oz	270	130
with lowfat milk	16 fl oz	220	70
with nonfat milk	16 fl oz	160	10
with soy milk	16 fl oz	150	70
Venti			
with whole milk	20 ft oz	350	160
with lowfat milk	20 fl oz	270	90
with nonfat milk	20 fl oz	200	10

with soy milk	20 fl oz	190	90
Caffe Mocha with whipping cream			
Short			
with whole milk	8 fl oz	250	150
with lowfat milk	8 ft oz	220	120
with nonfat milk	8 fl oz	200	100
Tall			
with whole milk	12 fl oz	340	190
with lowfat milk	12 fl oz	300	150
with nonfat milk	12 fl oz	260	100
Grande			
with whole milk	16 fl oz	410	220
with lowfat milk	16 fl oz	370	160
with nonfat milk	16 fl oz	320	110
Venti			
with whole milk	20 fl oz	500	250
with lowfat milk	20 fl oz	440	190
with nonfat milk	20 fl oz	380	120
Caffe Mocha (iced) with whipping cream			
Short			
with whole milk	8 fl oz	180	110
with iowfat milk	8 fl oz	170	90
with nonfat milk	8 fl oz	150	80
Tall			
with whole milk	12 fl oz	290	160
with lowfat milk	12 fl oz	260	130
with nonfat milk	12 fl oz	230	100
Grande			
with whole milk	16 fl oz	390	220
with lowfat milk	16 fl oz	50	180
with nonfat milk	16 ft oz	310	130
Caffe Rhumba			
Tall			
with lowfat milk	12 fl oz	250	45
Grande			
with lowfat milk	16 ft oz	330	60
Venti			
with lowfat milk	20 fl oz	410	70
Cappuccino			
Short			
with whole milk	8 fl oz	100	45

with lowfat milk	8 fl oz	80	25
with nonfat milk	8 fl oz	60	0
with soy milk	8 fl oz	50	25
Tall			
with whole milk	12 fl oz	140	60
with lowfat milk	12 fl oz	110	35
with nonfat milk	12 fl oz	80	0
with soy milk	12 fl oz	70	35
Grande			
with whole milk	16 fl oz	180	80
with lowfat milk	16 fl oz	140	45
with nonfat milk	16 fl oz	110	5
with soy milk	16 fl oz	100	50
Venti			
with whole milk	20 fl oz	200	90
with lowfat milk	20 fl oz	160	50
with nonfat milk	20 fl oz	120	5
with soy milk	20 fl oz	110	50
Espresso			
Solo	1 fl oz	5	0
Doppio	2 fl oz	10	0
Con Panna			
Solo	1 l oz	30	25
Dopplo	2 ft oz	35	25
Macchiato			
Solo			
with whole milk	1 fl oz	15	5
with lowfat milk	1fl oz	10	0
with nonfat milk	1 fl oz	10	0
Doppio			
with whole milk	2 fl oz	20	5
with lowfat milk	2 fl oz	15	0
with nonfat milk	2 fl oz	15	
Frappuccino			
Tall			
with lowfat milk	12 ft oz	200	25
Grande			
with lowfat milk	16 fl oz	270	35
Venti			
with lowfat milk	20 fl oz	340	45
Power Frappuccino			
Tall	12 fl oz	290	20

Grande	16 fl oz	350	25
Venti	20 fl oz	410	25
Power Mocha Frappuccino			
Tall	12 fl oz	320	25
Grande	16 fl oz	390	25
Venti	20 fl oz	460	30
Cocoa Drinks			
Cocoa with whipping cream			
Short			
with whole milk	8 fl oz	260	160
with lowfat milk	8 fl oz	230	130
with nonfat milk	8 fl oz	210	100
Tall			
with whole milk	12 fl oz	350	190
with lowfat milk	12 fl oz	310	150
with nonfat milk	12 fl oz	270	100
Grande			
with whole milk	16 fl oz	440	230
with lowfat milk	16 fl oz	390	170
with nonfat milk	16 fl oz	330	110
Venti			
with whole milk	20 fl oz	530	270
with lowfat milk	20 fl oz	460	200
with nonfat milk	20 fl oz	390	120
Tea Drinks			
Chai Tea Latte hot			
Short			
with whole milk	8 fl oz	160	60
with lowfat milk	8 fl oz	130	30
with nonfat milk	8 fl oz	110	0
Tall			
with whole milk	12 fl oz	220	80
with lowfat milk	12 fl oz	190	45
with nonfat milk	12 fl oz	150	0

APPENDIX XVI
Body Mass Index (BMI)

Height	19	20	21	22	23	24	25	26	27	28	29	30	31	32	33	34	35	36	37	38	39	40
4' 10"	91	96	100	105	110	115	119	124	129	134	138	143	148	153	158	162	167	172	177	181	186	191
4' 11"	94	99	104	409	114	119	124	128	133	138	143	148	153	158	163	168	173	178	183	188	193	198
5'	97	102	107	112	118	123	128	133	138	143	148	153	158	163	168	174	179	184	189	194	199	204
5' 1"	100	106	111	116	122	127	132	137	142	148	153	158	164	169	174	180	185	190	195	201	206	211
5' 2"	104	109	115	120	126	31	136	142	147	153	158	164	168	175	180	186	191	196	202	207	213	218
5' 3"	107	113	118	124	130	135	141	146	152	158	163	169	175	180	186	191	197	203	208	214	220	225
5' 4"	110	116	122	128	134	140	145	151	157	163	1269	174	180	186	192	197	204	209	215	221	227	232
5' 5"	114	120	126	132	138	144	150	156	162	168	174	180	186	192	198	204	210	216	222	228	234	240
5' 6"	118	124	130	136	142	148	155	161	167	173	179	186	192	198	204	210	216	223	229	235	241	247
5' 7"	121	127	134	1440	146	153	159	166	172	178	185	191	198	201	211	217	223	230	236	242	249	255
5' 8"	125	131	138	144	151	158	164	171	177	184	190	197	203	210	216	223	230	236	243	249	256	262
5' 9"	128	135	142	149	155	162	169	176	182	189	196	203	209	216	223	230	236	243	250	257	263	270
5' 10"	132	139	146	153	160	167	174	181	188	195	202	209	216	222	229	236	243	250	257	264	271	278
5' 11"	136	143	150	157	165	172	179	186	193	200	208	215	222	229	236	243	250	257	265	272	279	286
6'	140	147	154	162	169	177	184	191	199	206	213	221	228	235	242	250	258	265	272	279	287	294
6' 1"	144	151	159	166	174	182	189	197	204	212	219	227	235	242	250	257	265	272	280	288	295	302
6' 2"	148	155	163	171	179	186	194	202	210	218	225	233	241	249	256	264	272	280	287	295	303	311
6' 3"	152	160	168	176	184	192	200	208	216	224	232	240	248	256	264	272	279	287	295	303	311	319
6' 4"	156	164	172	180	189	197	205	213	221	230	238	246	254	263	271	279	287	295	304	312	320	328

To use this chart: Find you height in the left column. Move across that row toward the right to find your approximate weight. Then follow weight column up to find your BMI in the red bar at the top.

BMI = 703 x weight in pounds divided by (Height in Inches)^2

APPENDIX XVII

Glossary of Weights and Measurements

Abbreviations Used	
t	teaspoon
T	tablespoon
C	cup
oz	ounce
Common Household Measures	
1T = 3 t	1 pint = 2C
1C = 8 oz	2 pints = 1 quart
1C = 16 T	1 gallon = 2 quarts
Weights	
1 kg = 2.2 lbs.	
1 kg = 1000 g	
1 oz = 28.35 g	
1 lb = 453.6 g	
1 lb = 0.454 kg	

APPENDIX XVIII

LOW FAT RECIPES

SOUPS

MUSHROOM SOUP

INGREDIENTS: ½ pound fresh mushrooms, slices
2 t olive oil
2 cans (10 ¾ oz each) chicken or vegetable broth
2 T dry vermouth
1 t dry sherry
juice of 1 lemon (about ¼ C)
dash of Tabasco sauce

In a medium saucepan, sauté mushrooms in olive oil. Cook until just tender. Gently mix in chicken or vegetable broth. Add lemon juice, vermouth or sherry, and Tabasco sauce, and heat until hot.

Yield: 5 one-cup servings
Calories per serving: 90 Total; Fat: 13 g

CARROT SOUP

INGREDIENTS: 1 medium onion, chopped
3 small cloves garlic, minced
3 cloves
freshly ground black pepper to taste
1 t thyme
2 cans (10 ¾ oz each) chicken or vegetable broth
12 carrots, sliced (about 6 cups)
4 potatoes, peeled and cubed (about 4 cups)

In a soup pot or large casserole, combine onion, garlic, and thyme. Mix in carrots, potatoes, cloves and pepper. Add chicken or vegetable broth and enough water to cover vegetables. Bring soup to a boil. Reduce heat, cover, and simmer for minutes. Remove cloves. Remove 2 cups of carrots and potatoes and set aside. Puree soup in blender. Pour back into soup pot. Mix in reserved carrot-potato mixture.

Yield: 12 one-cup servings
Calories per serving: 69 Total; Fat: 0 g

CUCUMBER SOUP

INGREDIENTS: 2 cucumbers
2 C nonfat yogurt
1 can (10 ¾ oz) chicken or vegetable broth
1 clove garlic, crushed
coriander leaves for garnish

Peel cucumbers and grate. Spoon yogurt into a medium casserole and stir until smooth. Stir in chicken or vegetable broth. Mix in garlic. Squeeze grated cucumbers to take water out and add them to yogurt mixture. Add salt to taste. Chill in refrigerator for several hours. Garnish with coriander.

Yield: 5 one-cup servings
Calories per serving: 78 Total; Fat: 0 g

BEAN SOUP WITH SQUASH AND TOMATOES

INGREDIENTS: 2 C dried red kidney beans
1 medium zucchini, sliced into 1/2 – inch pieces
1 can (16 oz) chopped tomatoes, with juice
1 medium onion, minced
1 cup water
1 can chicken or vegetable broth (10 ¾ oz) defatted
3 cloves garlic, minced
1 t minced ginger root
½ t coriander powder
½ t cayenne pepper
1 t cumin
1 t turmeric

Cover beans with boiling water and let soak for 4 hours. Drain; add water to cover and cook 1 hour or until tender. Drain, remove about 7/8 of the beans and puree with chicken or vegetable broth in blender. Add puree back to the whole beans, set aside. In a large soup pot, sauté onion, garlic, and ginger root in olive oil. Add a splash of water and cook vegetables until soft. Mix in cumin, tumeric, coriander, and cayenne. Stir in bean mixture, zucchini, and spinach. Add tomatoes. If mixture is too thick, slowly add water, a few tablespoons at a time, until desired consistency is reached. Cook 5 minutes.

Yield: 10 one-cup servings
Calories per serving: 154 Total; Fat: 8 g

MINESTRONE SOUP

INGREDIENTS: ½ small onion
½ small carrot
1T spaghetti, macaroni or noodle
½ clove garlic
1 leaf cabbage
1 bay leaf
½ medium tomato
1t oil
1/8 t peppers
1 t salt (seasoning)
Garnish coriander leaves

Chop onion, shred cabbage and dice carrot fine. Heat oil in a saucepan, add onion and carrot saute. Add stock, bring to boil. Add macaroni, skinned and chopped tomato and bay leaf. Simmer gently for 20 minutes. Add the cabbage and seasoning. Cook until the vegetables are soft. Garnish with coriander leaves.

Yield: One serving; Serving Size: one bowl
Calories per serving: 80 Total; Fat: 1.5 g

CHICKEN SWEET CORN SOUP

INGREDIENTS: ½ lb chicken
2 C stock
small corn on the cob
1 ½ t cornflour
1T water
1 egg white or egg substitute
salt and pepper - to taste

Boil the chicken in stock for 20 minutes. Put the stock aside and shred the chicken. Grate the corn on the cob, add stock and cook for 20 minutes. Add shredded chicken mixture (keep some chicken shreds for garnishing) and bring to boil again. Make paste of cornflour with water and add the mixture to the soup and cook for 3 minutes, stirring constantly. Add salt and pepper and when the mixture is simmering, add the lightly beaten egg white or egg substitute. Stir with a fork in one direction to create "threads" of egg white. Pour soup into deep serving bowl and serve hot, garnished with chicken shreds.

Yield: One serving; Serving Size: one bowl
Calories per serving: 300 Total; Total Fat: 3 g

VEGETABLE SOUP

INGREDIENTS:

1 carrot, pared and diced
2 small zucchini, grated
2 onions, chopped
1 green bell pepper, diced
2 C cooked dal (lentil)
1 C cooked brown rice
1 C canned puree tomatoes
2 T olive oil
1 clove garlic, minced
3 C stock (meat or vegs for broth
2 C water
½ t oregano
½ t salt
½ t curry powder
1 T fresh coriander for garnishing

Heat oil; add onion, pepper, carrot, garlic and saute. Add zucchini and cook for an additional 7 minutes. Add stock or (chicken, broth), water, dal, tomatoes, and bay leaf. Bring to a boil over medium heat. Reduce heat to medium and simmer for 15 minutes. Add salt, pepper and simmer 10 minutes longer. Add rice, remove from heat and add lemon juice. Garnish with coriander leaves.

Yield: 5-6 servings; Serving Size: one bowl
Calories per serving: 190 Total; Total Fat: 3 g

SALADS

VEGETABLE SALAD

INGREDIENTS:

1 large cucumber, cubed
1 can (15 ½ oz) dark red kidney beans; drained and rinsed
2-3 carrots thinly sliced (3/4 cup)
1 tomato, coarsely chopped
¾ C red pepper, roasted or plain coarsely chopped
¾ C coarsely chopped red onion
½ C lemon juice
freshly ground pepper to taste
½ C fresh coriander

Combine all ingredients and mix so that vegetables are well covered. Refrigerate and chill or serve right away.

Yield: 6 one-cup servings; serving of size cups
Calories per cup: 105 Total; Fat: 12 g

SPINACH SALAD

INGREDIENTS: 1 package (10 oz) fresh spinach, washed and shredded
1 C sliced mushrooms
1 cucumber, peeled and sliced thin
1 carrot grated
10 water chestnuts, sliced
1 t olive oil
2 t soy sauce
3 T fresh lemon juice
3 green onions, sliced
1½ T honey
1 T pine nuts

In a salad bowl, combine spinach, water chestnuts, green onions, mushrooms, and cucumber slices. Mix together olive oil, soy sauce, lemon juice, and honey and pour over salad. Sprinkle with pine nuts.

Yield: 8 servings
Calories per serving: 55 Total; Total Fat: 20 g

BLACK BEAN AND CORN SALAD

INGREDIENTS: 4 C frozen corn
2 cans (15 oz each) black beans or other beans
1 C chopped red and/or green pepper
½ t salt (optional)
½ C white vinegar
½-1 t freshly ground black pepper
½-1 t chili powder
¼ C pickled jalapeno pepper (optional)

Cook corn until tender according to package directions. Drain and rinse beans and place in bowl or casserole. Mix in peppers. Drain cooked corn and add to bean mixture. Combine vinegar, salt, and spices and pour over corn and beans. Mix well. Cover and refrigerate several hours.

Yield: 12 half-cup servings
Calories per cup: 102 Total; Total fat: 10 g

RED POTATO SALAD

INGREDIENTS: 4-5 red potatoes
½ C nonfat yogurt
3 T low-fat mayonnaise
1 t Dijon mustard
1 t tarragon
1 T white vinegar
½ t salt (optional)

Scrub potatoes thoroughly. Steam until tender. Meanwhile, combine remaining ingredients. Set aside. Cut potatoes into chunks (do not remove skin). Pour sauce over potatoes so they are thoroughly coated. Serve warm or cold.

Yield: 6 servings
Calories per serving: 95 Total; Total Fat: 5 g

CORIANDER CHICKEN SALAD

INGREDIENTS: 6 boneless, skinless chicken breasts
2 C broccoli flowerets
½ C unbleached white flour
2 T low-fat mayonnaise
½ t salt (optional)
¼ t freshly ground black pepper
2 T nonfat yogurt
1 T mustard

Shake chicken with flour, salt, and pepper and cook. Bake at 375° for 20 minutes. Cut chicken into large chunks, mix with coriander, and set side. Steam broccoli until just tender. Combine mayonnaise, yogurt, and mustard. Mix dressing with chicken. Stir in broccoli until coated with dressing.

Yield: 8 servings
Calories per serving: 110 Total; Total fat: 12 g

CHICKEN AND BEAN SALAD

INGREDIENTS: 1 chicken breast, skinned, cooked and shredded
2 C cooked chick peas (you can use canned)
2 C cooked black-eyed peas
2 carrots, pared and sliced
3 T vegetable oil

2 T vinegar
2 T coriander, chopped
1 t sesame oil
1 t soy sauce (low sodium)
2 t shredded ginger
2 green chilies, chopped
1 small red onion, chopped

Mix all the ingredients together.

Yield: 6 servings; Serving Size: one bowl
Calories per serving: 293 Total; Total Fat: 11 g

BEAN AND BROCCOLI SALAD

INGREDIENTS: 3 C broccoli flowers, cooked crisp
2 C cooked black-eyed peas
1/3 C diced roasted red pepper
2 T olive oil
1 T fresh lemon juice
2 T chopped coriander
2 chopped green chilies (if desired)
salt to taste

Stir all ingredients together in a bowl.

Yield: 2 servings; Serving Size: one bowl
Calories per serving: 419 Total; Total Fat: 15 g

OAT SALAD

INGREDIENTS: 1 C cooked oat groats
½ C cooked red kidney beans
½ C minced fresh coriander
¼ C fresh lemon juice
2 scallions, chopped finely
2 T olive oil
2 T minced fresh mint
2 green chillies cut into small pieces salt to taste

Stir all ingredients together.

Yield: 4 servings; Serving Size: one bowl
Calories per serving: 137 Total; Total Fat: 8 g

VEGETABLES

CAULIFLOWER SAUTE

INGREDIENTS: 2 C cauliflower flowerets
1 small onion, sliced (about ¼ cup)
1 t olive oil
1 t cumin seeds
½ t black pepper
salt to taste

Steam cauliflower until just tender. Set aside. In large skillet, sauté onion in olive oil until soft and golden. Add cumin seeds. Add steamed cauliflower, black pepper and salt.

Yield: 6 servings
Calories per serving: 37 Total; Total fat: 7 g

MIX VEGETABLES

INGREDIENTS: 2 zucchini, sliced (about 2 cups)
3 C combined red, yellow, green peppers, sliced
1 onion, sliced
1 clove garlic, minced
12 cloves
1 t thyme, oregano, or basil or combination
2 t olive oil
salt to taste

In a large skillet, sauté garlic cloves and onion in olive oil. Add cooked vegetables cook until tender. Stir in peppers, zucchini, salt, and herbs. Cover, cook until tender.

Yield: 8 servings
Calories per serving: 27 Total; Total fat: 10 g

SPINACH

INGREDIENTS: 10 ounces fresh spinach, washed and chopped
1 t ginger root shredded
1 t olive oil

In a large skillet, lightly sauté spinach in oil until soft. Stir in ginger and salt.

Yield: 4 servings
Calories per serving: 30 Total; Total fat: 10 g

CURRIED POTATOES AND PEAS

INGREDIENTS: 4 C peeled and cubed baking potatoes
1 C frozen peas
2 C sliced carrots
1 C coarsely chopped tomato
½ C chopped onion
pepper (optional)
1 t olive oil
½ C water
¼ t cayenne
1 t turmeric
½ t coriander
½ t cumin

In a large saucepan or casserole, sauté onions in olive oil until soft. Stir in tomato and spices. Add ½ cup water. Mix in potatoes until well covered with sauce and bring to a boil. Reduce heat, cover and simmer for about 10 minutes, stirring occasionally. Remove cover, add peas, and continue cooking until carrots and potatoes are tender.

Yield: 14 half-cup servings
Calories per serving: 31 Total; Total fat: 3 g

OKRA

INGREDIENTS: ½ C okra
1 small onion
1 t oil
¼ t turmeric powder
⅛ t red chili powder
⅛ t coriander powder
¼ t salt

Wash and dry or wipe okra with a wet cloth. Cut them into half-inch slice and slice the onion into long thin pieces. Heat oil in a teflon pan, gently put in the bhindis. Cook open stirring occasionally. When half done and less sticky, add onions and seasoning. Stir, cook covered on a slow fire until done and crisp.

Yield: One serving; Serving Size: one bowl
Calories per serving: 105 Total; Total Fat: 4.6 g

CURRIED CARROTS

INGREDIENTS: 2 medium size carrots, cut into small pieces
1 small green chili, cut into small pieces
1t oil
⅛ t cumin seeds
½ t grated ginger
pinch salt
pinch pepper

Heat oil, add cumin seeds, green chili, ginger and saute for 5 minutes. Add carrots, stir, let mixture stay on low heat about 10 to 15 minutes.

Yield: One serving; Serving Size: one bowl
Calories per serving: 80 Total; Total Fat: 4.6 g

CURRIED RED KIDNEY BEANS

INGREDIENTS: 1 3/4 C red kidney beans
1 ½ C chopped tomatoes (without skin)
3/4 t grated ginger
2 t Chili powder
1 T minced ginger
½ t minced garlic
1 t coriander powder
1 t cumin powder
3/4 t turmeric powder
3/4 t garam masalla
2 T chopped coriander leaves
2 T vegetable oil
2 T chopped coriander leaves
2 C finely sliced onions
1 t grated garlic
salt to taste

Wash and soak the rajmah over night. Add ½ teaspoon of baking soda. Wash rajmah thoroughly. Put rajmah, salt, red chili, ginger and garlic in 4 cups of water. Pressure cook the rajmah for 45 minutes or cook a crock pot. Then let it cool and drain the rajmah and reserve the stock separately. Grind onion to fine paste and fry it in heated oil until brown. Add turmeric powder and coriander powder. Fry for 10 minutes. Add skinned tomato pieces. Add the drained kidney beans and fry for another five minutes. Add rajmah masala. Add reserved stock and cook for 20 minutes until gravy thickens. Garnish with chopped coriander leaves. *You can add Binodrops to the curry to avoid possible discomfort due to gas.*

Yield: 6-8 servings; Serving Size: one bowl
Calories per serving: 376 Total; Total Fat: 5 g

STUFFED TOMATO

INGREDIENTS: 2 firm tomato
1 small potato
1 carrot
½ C peas
½ onions
2 T low fat cheese
¼ t red chili powder
¼ t garam masala
2 t oil
1 t fat
A sprig chopped coriander leaves
½ t salt

Cut off a thin slice of tomato from top and keep it aside. Scoop out the pulp and keep it aside. Drain off tomatoes and sprinkle a little salt into the cavities. Boil, peel and cut potato and carrot into small pieces. Chop onions fine. Heat oil, fry onions lightly. Add tomato pulp, cooked vegetables, paneer and seasoning. Cook till well mixed and a little dry. Add coriander leaves and remove from fire. Fill the tomato sheets with this mixture. Replace the tomato caps. Bake in a very moderate oven (325°F) for about 5-7 minutes. (Brush pan with a little oil before baking).

Yield: One serving; Serving Size: 2 tomatoes
Calories per serving: 288 Total; Total Fat: 5.5 g

EGGPLANT (BAINGAN) BHARTHA

INGREDIENTS: 1 small eggplant
1 small onion
1 small tomato
1 small green chili
1 t oil
½ t ginger, minced
¼ t red chili powder
¼ t garam masala
½ t salt
a sprig green coriander (chopped)

Broil the eggplant, peel, wash and mash well. Chop onion, tomato and green chili. Fry the onions lightly and add tomatoes, green chili and seasoning. Add the mashed eggplant and cook until dry and glossy. Serve hot, garnished with coriander leaves.

Yield: One serving; Serving Size: one bowl
Calories per serving: 187 Total; Total Fat: 5 g

PEAS AND CABBAGE

INGREDIENTS:
½ C peas
¼ cabbage of medium size
2 t ginger
⅛ t red chili powder (optional)
¼ t turmeric powder
1 green chili
1 T oil
⅛ t garam masala
A few coriander leaves
½ t salt

Chop ginger, shred cabbage. Fry ginger until golden brown. Add salt, red chili powder, turmeric and green chili. Fry lightly and add cabbage and peas. Cook lightly, stirring occasionally for 2 - 3 minutes and then cover. Sprinkle chopped coriander leaves and garam masala.

Yield: One serving; Serving Size: one bowl
Calories per serving: 212 Total; Total Fat: 5 g

MEATS

GINGER CHICKEN

INGREDIENTS:
5 boneless, skinless chicken breasts
2 cloves garlic, minced
1 t ground ginger
2 t minced ginger root
2 T cornstarch
1 t red pepper
1 ¼ C water
1 t ground fennel
3 T soy sauce
2 T olive oil

Cut chicken into bite-size pieces, sprinkle with ground ginger, and set aside for 15 minutes. Make a smooth paste of the cornstarch and 2 tablespoons of the water. Stir in 2 more tablespoons of water and soy sauce. Set aside. Sauté chicken in oil until cooked through. Stir in garlic, ginger root, red pepper and ground fennel. Mix in soy sauce mixture and heat until the sauce thickens. If sauce is too thick, add remaining water, ¼ cup at a time, until desired consistency is achieved. Stir in green onions and serve over rice.

Yield: 6 servings
Calories per serving: 172 Total; Total fat: 51 g

TANDORRI CHICKEN

INGREDIENTS: 4 boneless, skinless chicken breasts
¾ C nonfat yogurt
1 clove garlic, minced
½ T sliced ginger root
⅛ t cardamom
1 t paprika
⅛ t coriander
1 t ground fennel
1 ½ T lemon juice
1 T olive oil
¼ t black pepper
¼ t salt

Combine all ingredients except chicken (may be done in food processor) and pour over chicken breasts. Marinate in refrigerator for at least 24 hours. Place chicken with marinade in a shallow baking pan. Bake at 375°F for 30-45 minutes or until chicken is fully cooked.

Yield: 4 servings
Calories per serving: 77 Total; Total Fat: 20 g

CHICKEN BROCHETTES

INGREDIENTS: 6 boneless, skinless chicken breasts
½ t ginger powder
¼ C soy sauce
½ t fennel powder
½ C dry white wine or vermouth
1 clove garlic, minced

Cut chicken breasts into 1-inch cubes and place in a bowl or casserole. Combine soy sauce, wine, and garlic and pour over chicken. Marinate in refrigerator for at least 30 minutes. Preheat oven to broil or prepare grill. Remove chicken from marinade and reserve marinade. Skewer chicken and broil or grill until cooked through, basting occasionally with marinade. Heat marinade and pour over chicken.

Yield: 6 servings
Calories per serving: 160 Total; Total Fat: 20 g

CHICKEN WITH SPINACH

INGREDIENTS: 3-pound chicken, skinned and cut
2 C chopped spinach (or 2 packages frozen cut spinach)
4 tomatoes, chopped
2 T oil
2 onions, sliced thin
4 garlic cloves, minced
1-inch cinnamon stick
2 t minced fresh ginger
2 t coriander seeds

Boil the chicken until tender. Remove chicken and reserve stock. Heat the oil in a wok or frying pan, saute the onions and garlic until light brown. Add the minced ginger, coriander seeds, and saute 2 minutes. Add the chicken pieces and saute 5 more minutes, turning chicken on all sides. Add the tomatoes, the spinach, and one half of the chicken stock. Cover and simmer for 20 minutes.

Yield: 4 servings; Serving Size: one bowl
Calories per serving: 250 Total; Total Fat: 5.5 g

CHICKEN WITH APRICOTS

INGREDIENTS: 1 3-pound chicken, skinned and cut
4 apricots, pits removed, chopped
4 tomatoes, chopped
2 onions, sliced thin
2 green chilies
2 garlic cloves
1 t cumin seeds
2 T oil
½ C water
2 T chopped coriander leaves
salte to taste

Grind chilies, garlic and cumin seeds, making into a paste. In a wok, saute onions until golden. Add the chicken pieces and saute over medium heat until chicken is brown, about 15 minutes. Add the masala paste, tomatoes, apricots and salt, plus ½ cup of water. Simmer until meat is tender, 15-20 minutes.

Yield: 4 servings; Serving Size: 2 pieces
Calories per serving: 220 Total; Total Fat: 5.5 g

CHICKEN WITH CABBAGE

INGREDIENTS: 1 3-pound chicken, skinned and cut
1 small cabbage, shredded
2 T oil
2 T coriander leaves
2 onions, chopped fine
1 T ginger/garlic paste
½ t red pepper
1 t salt

Boil the chicken in covered water until tender. Remove chicken and reserve stock. Wash and shred the cabbage. In a wok or heavy skillet, heat the oil and lightly saute the onions, garlic, ginger paste and pepper. Stir in the cabbage and the salt. Cook until cabbage is half-way crisp. Add the chicken pieces and the stock and heat through, 5 to 10 minutes.

Yield: 4 servings; Serving Size: one bowl
Calories per serving: 230 Total; Total Fat: 5.5 g

BUTTERMILK CHICKEN

INGREDIENTS: 2 pieces tandari chicken
2 Peeled tomatoes, pureed (or small pureed can)
1 t oil
1 small onion, finely chopped
1 t ginger, grated
2 T low fat butter milk
2 cloves garlic
¼ t garam masala
½ t red chili powder
1 ½ t sugar
¼ t salt

Heat oil, fry onions, ginger, and garlic. Add red chili powder, tomato puree, salt and sugar. Cook on slow fire. Put in blender. Lightly Fry the pieces of tandoori chicken and remove from fat. Remove pan from heat and add tomato sauce (as cooked above) and cook for about 5 minutes. Add buttermilk. Mix it, cook for

5 minutes. Add the fried chicken. Simmer for 10 minutes or until the flavor of the sauce penetrates. Remove from heat. Sprinkle with roasted ground black cumin seed, garam masala and finely chopped coriander leaves.

Yield: One serving; Serving Size: 2 pieces or 1 joint
Calories per serving: 400 Total; Total Fat: 20 g

SEEKH KABABS (Turkey)

INGREDIENTS: ¼ lb ground turkey
1 t lime juice
¼ t poppy seeds
1 clove
3 pepper corns
1 t grated ginger
1 almond
a pinch nutmeg
½ t cumin seeds
¼ t water
¼ t low fat yoghurt
⅛ t red chilli powder
⅛ t garam masala
1 t coriander seeds
a few coriander leaves
¼ t salt

Add salt and lime juice to meat and set aside for one hour to allow the mince to become tender. Roast poppy seeds, almond, cumin seeds, cloves, coriander seeds and pepper corns on a griddle. Grind these with ginger, nutmeg and add low fat yoghurt. Mix with minced meat, add red chilli powder and garam masala. Add water and knead hard for a few minutes as this makes the paste stickey and suitable for holding on the skewers. Chop coriander leaves finely and add to the paste. Divide into 4 long sections and flatten them. Pass skewer through the center of each part, and using a hand, fold the meat on to it. Rotate the skewer slowly and press the meat gently with fingers, moistened with a little water, until it completely circles the skewer. Leave for 10 minutes and roast on a charcoal fire or in an oven. Turn slowly when one side is done. Do not turn too frequently. Grill until the kababs they are evenly browned on all sides.

Yield: One serving; Serving Size: 4 kababs
Calories per serving: 200 Total; Total Fat: 10 g
Cholesterol: 75 mg; Fiber: 0.2 g

CURRIED GROUND TURKEY

INGREDIENTS: ½ lb ground turkey
2 peeled, chopped tomatoes
½ C peas
1 T oil
1 clove
¼ t turmeric
½ stick cinnamon
1 t ginger
1 brown cardamon
2 cloves garlic
1 small onion
⅛ t chili powder
2 T water
1 bay leaf
½ (finely cut) green chilli
½ t salt
a sprig coriander leaves

Roast clove, cinnamon and cardamon. Remove immediately from heat and crush. Heat oil and fry the onions until golden brown. Remove from the heat, add red chili powder and a teaspoon of hot water. Place on slow heat and cook until water is absorbed. Add the turkey, bay leaves, crushed whole spices, salt and turmeric. Cover, stirring occasionally until the juices in the mince dries up. Grind ginger and garlic, add to the mince and cook for about 5 minutes. Add blanched, peeled and chopped tomatoes. Cover and cook until the tomatoes are mixed up with the mince, and gravy thickens. Add peas and fry for a few minutes. Add water. Return to heat and simmer until done.

Yield: One serving; Serving Size: one bowl
Calories per serving: 300 Total; Total Fat: 10 g

FISH

BAKED FISH WITH MINT

INGREDIENTS: 1 ½ pounds fish fillets
1 can (16 oz) tomatoes, chopped, juice reserved
4 T mint (mince in blend)
¾ C chopped onion
1 t chopped red or green chili pepper
2 cloves garlic, minced

1 t minced ginger
1 t olive oil
1 tablespoon fresh lemon juice
salt to taste (optional)

Preheat oven to 375°F. In a medium skillet, sauté onion, ginger and garlic in olive oil. Cook until soft. Mix in cornstarch. Add tomatoes and their juice and minced mint and mix until well blended. Cook over medium-high heat until sauce thickens. Add chili pepper. Spoon half the sauce into a baking pan large enough to hold fillets in one layer. Place fillets over sauce. Salt fillets and sprinkle with lemon juice. Cover fillets with remaining sauce and bake for 20 minutes or until they flake easily.

Yield: 6 servings
Calories per serving: 150 Total; Total Fat: 18 g

SALMON SOUFFLE

INGREDIENTS: 1 can (8 oz) salmon
3 egg whites
1 C skim milk
1 C fine bread crumbs of 2 slices whole-wheat bread
½ t black pepper and salt to taste

Preheat oven to 350°F. Grease a small casserole with margarine. Prepare salmon by carefully rinsing it with water and removing any bones. Set aside. Heat skim milk and bread crumbs slowly in a double boiler until thick. Meanwhile, whip egg whites until stiff but not dry. Set aside. Flake salmon with a fork and add it to the thickened milk mixture. Remove from heat. Fold salmon mixture into egg whites. Pour into casserole and bake for 30 minutes.

Yield: 4 servings
Calories per serving: 149 Total; Total Fat: 32 g

SWEET AND SOUR SHRIMP

INGREDIENTS: 1 lb precooked shrimp
2 large carrots
1 green pepper, sliced
1 red pepper, sliced
¾ C sliced onion
3 green onions
2 t ginger root, minced

2 T brown sugar
2 t garlic, minced
4 T white vinegar
¼ C tomato sauce
¼ C water
2 t cornstarch
4 T water
2 t soy sauce
2 cloves garlic, minced or pressed

Combine brown sugar, vinegar, tomato sauce, water, cornstarch, soy sauce, garlic, and ginger. Set aside. Lay both carrots on cutting board and slice each lengthwise at 1/8-ince intervals. Cut these strips into pieces 1 ½ - 2 inches long. You should have about 2 cups of strips. Slice green onions in half and cut into 1-inch pieces. Set aside. In a wok or large skillet, sauté carrots and onion in olive oil. Mix for a few seconds. Add 1 tablespoon water and mix for a minute or two. Add 3 more tablespoons water and cover the pan. Cook for a minute or two. Mix in shrimp, peppers, and green onions. Add sauce. Cover to let steam cook shrimp. Uncover occasionally to stir shrimp. Add 1 tablespoon water. Cook until shrimp have changed color and are opaque.

Yield: 5 servings
Calories per serving: 167 Total; Total Fat: 21 g

SHRIMP CURRY

INGREDIENTS: 1 pound shrimps
3 cloves garlic
2 onions
½ t salt
1 tamarind (cleaned and washed)
2 t oil
½ t cumin seeds
¼ C water
½ t mustard seeds
a few sprigs coriander
2-3 peppercorns
a few curry leaves

Except for the shrimp and curry leaves, grind all of the above ingredients together. Heat oil, fry curry leaves, add ground masala and fry well. When brown in color, add shrimp. Lightly fry, adding water and continue cooking until done.

Yield: One serving; Serving Size: one bowl
Calories per serving: 172 Total; Total Fat: 9 g

DESSERTS

PUMPKIN CAKE

INGREDIENTS: 1 ¼ C unbleached white flour
½ C rye flour
1 C pumpkin puree
¼ C skim milk
1 egg, plus 1 egg white
¾ C brown sugar
½ C raisins
1 t baking soda
1 t baking powder
6 T margarine
½ t salt
1 ½ t cinnamon
1 t cardamom

Preheat oven to 350°F. Grease a loaf pan with margarine and lightly flour. Combine flours, baking soda, baking powder, salt, cinnamon, cardamom, and raisins. Set aside. In a large mixing bowl, mix together pumpkin puree, brown sugar, and margarine. Add skim milk, egg, and egg white and mix until smooth. Stir in flour mixture. Pour batter into loaf pan and bake for 45-60 minutes or until a cake tester comes out clean.

Yield: 18 half-inch slices
Calories per slice: 128 Total; Total Fat: 34 g

LEMON LOAF

INGREDIENTS: ½ C sugar
½ C applesauce
grated rind of 1 lemon
2 C unbleached white flour
¾ C buttermilk
3 T sugar
2 T fresh lemon juice
¼ C fresh lemon juice
1 t baking soda
¼ t salt
2 t baking powder

Preheat oven to 375oF. Grease a loaf pan with margarine. Mix together flour, slat, baking powder, and baking soda and set aside. In a large mixing bowl, mix

½ cup sugar and applesauce. Add grated lemon peel and mix until smooth. Add flour mixture to applesauce mixture alternately with buttermilk mixture. Do not overmix. Pour into loaf pan and bake for 30-45 minutes or until a cake tester comes out clean. Let cool in pan 10 minutes. In a small saucepan, combine 2 tablespoons lemon juice and 3 tablespoons sugar and stir over low heat until sugar dissolves. Pierce top of cake with fork or skewer. Spoon lemon-sugar mixture into holes. Let cool for easy slicing.

Yield: 10 slices
Calories per slice: 150 Total; Total Fat: 1 g

ORANGE CAKE

INGREDIENTS:
1 ½ C unbleached white flour
½ C sugar
2 t baking powder
½ C orange juice
¼ t salt
3 egg whites
½ C applesauce
2 T orange juice

Preheat oven to 350°F. Grease a loaf pan with margarine. Combine flour, baking powder, and salt. Set aside. In a large mixing bowl, beat applesauce and sugar. Add flour mixture, alternating with ½ cup orange juice, until batter is smooth. In another bowl, whip egg whites until stiff but not dry. Fold egg whites into batter. Pour batter into loaf pan and bake for 40-50 minutes or until a cake tester comes out clean. Cool in pan for 10 minutes. Poke holes in top of cake. Pour 2 tablespoons orange juice into holes.

Yield: 10 slices
Calories per slice: 119 Total; Total Fat: 2 g

CINNAMON SUGAR COFFEE CAKE

INGREDIENTS:
1 ½ C unbleached white flour
1 t cinnamon
½ C applesauce
1 t baking soda
1 ½ t baking powder
1 cup nonfat yogurt
1 egg plus 1 egg white
½ t salt
¼ C brown sugar

1 t vanilla
¾ C sugar

Preheat oven to 350°F. Grease an 8-inch springform pan with margarine. Combine flour, baking powder, baking soda, and salt in a bowl. Set aside. In small bowl combine ¼ cup brown sugar, ¼ cup of the granulated sugar, and cinnamon and set aside. In a large mixing bowl, mix remaining ½ cup sugar with applesauce. Add egg and egg white and vanilla and mix until batter is smooth. Add flour and yogurt alternately and mix until batter is smooth. Pour batter into springform pan. Pour sugar mixture on top of batter and, with a knife, swirl sugar into batter. Bake for 35-50 minutes or until cake tester comes out clean.

Yield: 8 slices
Calories per slice: 210 Total; Total Fat: 7 g

CINNAMON SWEET CAKES

INGREDIENTS:
¾ C whole-wheat flour
¼ C applesauce
¾ C unbleached white flour
1 egg
½ C skim milk
2 t baking powder
½ C sugar
½ t salt

Topping:
½ C brown sugar
1/3 C coarsely chopped walnuts
1 t cinnamon
1 T margarine
1 T unbleached white flour

Preheat oven to 375°F. Grease an 8x8 –inch baking pan with margarine. In a large bowl, beat together applesauce, egg, and skim milk. Add sugar, whole-wheat flour, white flour, baking powder, and salt and beat until smooth. Spoon batter into baking pan. (batter will be thick). To make topping, combine brown sugar, walnuts, flour, and cinnamon in a small bowl. Melt margarine and stir into mixture. Sprinkle topping over batter. Bake for about 25 minutes or until cake tester comes out clean.

Yield: 16 square
Calories per square: 120 Total; Total Fat: 20 g

BUTTERMILK POUND CAKE

INGREDIENTS:
1 ¾ C cake flour
¾ C nonfat buttermilk
¾ C sugar
1 egg + 2 egg whites
½ t baking soda
1 t baking powder

½ t vanilla
¼ t salt
¼ t almond extract
½ C margarine

Preheat oven to 375°F and greese an 8-inch springform pan with margarine. Combine flour, baking soda, baking powder, and salt and set aside. In an electric mixer, cream margarine and sugar. Add egg and egg whites, vanilla, and almond extract and mix until smooth. Add flour mixture and buttermilk and mix until smooth. Pour into springform pan and bake for 30-40 minutes or until cake tester comes out clean. When cool, frost it with our number-one favorite choice, Don Mauer's Fantastic Fudge Frosting (page 262).

Yield: 12 slices
Calories per slice: 160 Total ; Fat: 64 g
With Don Mauer's Frosting, Calories 245; Fat: 68 g

BANANA CAKE

INGREDIENTS: 1 C whole-wheat flour
½ C unbleached white flour
¾ C wheat germ
3 ripe bananas, mashed
1 egg
5 prunes, chopped
½ C applesauce
½ C brown sugar
1 t cinnamon
¾ t vanilla
½ t grated nutmeg
2 t baking powder
¼ t baking soda
¼ t salt

Preheat oven to 350oF. Grease a loaf pan with margarine. Mix flours, wheat germ, cinnamon, nutmeg, baking powder, baking soda, and salt and set aside. In an electric mixer, mix applesauce and brown sugar. Add vanilla and egg and mix well. Add bananas and blend until smooth. Mix in flour mixture. Fold in prunes. Pour batter into loaf pan and bake for 40-60 minutes or until a cake tester comes out clean.

Yield: 10 slices
Calories per slice: 166 Total; Total Fat: 6 g

APPLE CAKE

INGREDIENTS: 4 C delicious apples, peeled and cut into chunks
¾ C unbleached white flour
1 C whole-wheat flour
¾ C brown sugar
½ C applesauce
1 egg
1 egg white
1 t vanilla
1 ½ t cinnamon
1 t baking soda
¼ t grated nutmeg
½ t salt

Preheat oven to 350oF. Grease an 8-inch springform pan with margarine and dust with flour. In an electric mixer, beat together brown sugar and applesauce. Add vanilla, egg, and egg white and beat until smooth. Add flours, salt, baking soda, cinnamon, and nutmeg and beat until smooth. With a large (wooden) spoon or rubber spatula, mix in apples. The batter will be very sticky and stiff. Spoon batter into pan and bake for 40-60 minutes or until a cake tester comes out clean.

Yield: 10 slices
Calories per slice: 189 Total; Total Fat: 6 g

ORANGE SOUFFLE

INGREDIENTS: cooking spray
¼ C fresh orange juice
2 t grated orange rind
1 T sugar
3 T all-purpose flour
¾ C 1% low-fat milk
¼ C sugar
5 large egg whites (at room temperature)
¼ t cream of tartar
2 T sugar
1 t powdered sugar
dash of salt

Preheat oven to 375°. Coat a 1 ½- quart souffle dish with cooking spray. Sprinkle with 1 tablespoon sugar. Set aside. Place flour in a small saucepan. Gradually add milk, stirring with a whisk until blended. Add 1/4 cup sugar and rind. Stir well. Bring to a boil over medium heat. Cook for one minute or until thickened, stirring constantly. Stir in juice and set aside. Beat egg whites, cream of tartar, and salt at high speed with electric mixer until soft peaks form. Gradually add 2 tablespoons sugar, 1 tablespoon at a time, beating until stiff peaks form. Gently fold one-fourth egg white mixture into orange mixture; gently fold in remaining egg white mixture. Spoon into prepared souffle dish and bake at 375° for 40 minutes or until puffy and set. Sprinkle with powdered sugar. Serve immediately.

Yield: 4 servings; Serving Size: one cup
Calories per serving: 150 Total; Total Fat: 1 g

CAPPUCCINO PUDDING CAKE

INGREDIENTS: 1 C all-purpose flour
2/3 C sugar
2 T unsweetened cocoa
2 t baking powder
½ C evaporated skim milk
1 t vegetable oil
1 t vanilla extract
¼ C semisweet chocolate morsels
1 C firmly packed dark brown sugar
¼ C unsweetened cocoa
1 ¾ C hot water
2 (.77-ounce) envelopes instant cappuccino coffee mix or
1/4 cup other instant flavored coffee mix
9 T frozen vanilla yogurt

Preheat oven to 350°. Combine first 5 ingredients in a 9-inch square baking pan, and stir well. Add milk, oil, and vanilla, stirring until smooth. Stir in chocolate morsels. Combine brown sugar and 1/4 cup cocoa and sprinkle over batter. Combine water and coffee mix, stirring to dissolve. Pour coffee mixture over batter; do not stir. Bake at 350° for 40 minutes or until cake springs back when touched lightly in center. Serve warm with 1 tablespoon frozen yogurt.

Yield: 9 servings; Serving Size: one bowl
Calories per serving: 247 Total; Total Fat: 3 g

RICE PUDDING

INGREDIENTS: ½ C rice
2 quarts low-fat (2%) milk
1 T ground cardamon
½ C raisins
2 T sliced skinless almond

½ C sugar
few drops of rose water (optional)

Wash the rice and let soak in water for 1 hour. Bring the milk to a boil and add the rice. Stir gently until the mixture thickens a bit, and then reduce heat. Add the ground cardamon, raisins and sugar, and the rose water, if used. Stir gently a few minutes until the mixture gets thick and creamy. Add almonds and serve.

Yield: 6 servings; Serving Size: one cup
Calories per serving: 240 Total; Total Fat: 4.7 g

APRICOT MOUSSE

INGREDIENTS: 1 lb dried apricots
½ C sugar
¼ C cool whip
½ t vanilla
2 T lemon juice
toasted flaxed brown almonds

Soak the apricots in water and lemon juice for 12-24 hours. Simmer until tender. Sieve or liquidize and sweeten with sugar. Fold in with whipped cream. Chill. Spoon into small bowl and top with flaked browned almonds.

Yield: 6 servings; Serving Size: one bowl
Calories per serving: 100 Total; Total Fat: 0 g

MANDARIN YOGURT DESSERT

INGREDIENTS: 1 bowl cool whip - medium size
4 low-fat orange mandarin yogurt
2 cans mandarin segments

Drain mandarin segments and mix well with yogurt and cool whip.

Yield: 8 servings; Serving Size: one bowl
Calories per serving: 225 Total; Total Fat: 2.6 g

PEACH CRUMB CAKE

INGREDIENTS: 2 C sliced fresh peaches
1/3 C graham cracker crumbs
½ t ground cinnamon

vegetable cooking spray
1/8 t ground nutmeg
2 t reduced-calorie margarine, melted

Arrange peach slices in bottom of an 8-inch square baking dish coated with cooking spray. Combine graham cracker crumbs, cinnamon, and nutmeg in a small bowl, stirring well. Add margarine, and stir until blended. Sprinkle graham cracker crumb mixture over peaches, and bake at 350o for 30 minutes. Serve warm.

Yield: 4 servings; Serving Size: ½ cup
Calories per service: 75 Total; Total Fat: 2 g

CHEESECAKE

INGREDIENTS: 2 ½ C 1% low-fat cottage cheese
2 t unflavored gelatin
¼ C sugar
14 (2 1/2 –inch) graham cracker squares, crushed
2 T cold water
⅛ t almond extract
⅓ C Sugar
6 drops red food coloring (optional)
1 t vanilla extract
1 (16-ounce) can cherries in water
¼ C reduced-calorie margarine melted
2 t cornstarch

Sprinkle gelatin over cold water in a small sauce and let stand 1 minute. Cook over low heat, stirring constantly, 2 minutes or until gelatin dissolves. Let cool. Add sugar to equal 1/3 cup sugar to cooled gelatin. Combine cottage cheese and vanilla in container of an electric blender; cover and process until smooth. Gradually add gelatin mixture to cottage cheese mixture. Place cottage cheese mixture in a bowl, and chill 10 to 20 minutes or until slightly thickened, stirring occasionally. Drain cherries, reserving liquid. Combine cornstarch and cherry liquid in a small saucepan; stir until smooth. Cook over medium heat, stirring constantly, until cornstarch mixture comes to a boil. Reduce heat, and cook 1 minute. Remove from heat, and stir in cherries. Let cherry mixture cool slightly; add sugar substitute to equal ¼ cup sugar, almond extract, and red food coloring, if desired. Set cherry mixture aside.

Yield: 4 servings; Serving size: one slice
Calories per serving: 150 Total; Total Fat: 4 g

STRAWBERRY MOUSSE

INGREDIENTS: 1 ½ C sliced fresh strawberries
1 (0.3-ounce) package sugar-free strawberry-flavored gelatin
2/3 C instant nonfat dry milk powder
½ C water
6 ice cubes

Combine gelatin and water in a small saucepan, stirring well; let stand 1 minute. Cook over low heat, stirring constantly, 1 minute or until gelatin dissolves. Combine gelatin mixture, strawberries, and milk powder in container of an electric blender; cover and process until smooth. Add ice cubes, one at a time, processing until blended. Spoon mixture evenly into 6 parfait glasses. Cover and chill.

Yield: 6 servings; Serving Size: ½ cup
Calories per serving: 45 Total; Total Fat: trace

Sources: *Healthy Heart South Asian Diet Eater's Choice Low Fat Cookbook*

APPENDIX XIX

LIST OF ABBREVIATIONS

ACTH	Adrenocorticotropic Hormone
ADA	American Dietetic Association
AHA	American Heart Association
AHI	Apnea-hypopnea Index
AHRQ	Agency for Health Care Research and Quality
ALT	Alanine Transaminase
AMA	Antimitochondrial Antibody
ANA	Antinuclear Antibody
AOA	American Obesity Association
AST	Aspartate Transaminase
ATP	Adenosine Triphosphate
BEE	Basal Energy Expenditure
BMI	Body Mass Index
BMR	Basal Metabolic Rate
BPD	Biliopancreatic Diversion
CBC	Complete Blood Count
CDC	Centers for Disease Control
CNS	Central Nervous System
COPD	Chronic Obstructive Pulmonary Disease
CPAP	Continuous Positive Airway Pressure
CT	Computed Tomography
CTS	Carparal Tunnel Syndrome
CVD	Cardiovascular Disease
CVI	Chronic Venous Insufficiency
DHEAH	Diethylaminoethoxlhexestrol
DJD	Degenerative Joint Disease
DVT	Deep Vein Thrombosis
EC	Endometrial Cancer
ESD	End Stage Renal Disease
ESRD	End Stage Renal Disease
FDA	Food and Drug Administration
GI	Glycemic Index
HCV	Hepatitis C Virus
HDL	High Density Lipoprotein
HFCS	High Fructose Corn Syrup
HSP	Hemorrhagic Stroke Project
HSS	Health and Human Services
HT	Human Transporter (receptor)
HTN	Hypertension
IBW	Ideal Body Weight

IOM	Institute of Medicine
IR	Insulin Resistance
IRS	Insulin Resistance Syndrome
IU	International Unit
IV	Intravenous
LDL	Low Density Lipoprotein
LFT	Liver Function Tests
MAO	Monoamine Oxide
MI	Myocardial Infarction
MRI	Magnetic Resonance Imagery
MSG	Monosodium Glutamate
MSLT	Multiple Sleep Latency Test
MWT	Maintenance of Wakefulness Test
NAFLD	Non-Alcoholic Fatty Liver Diseases
NASH	Non Alcoholic Hepatic Steatosis and Steatohepatitis
NCHS	National Center for Health Statistics
NE	Norepinephrine
NHANES	National Health and Nutrition Examination Survey
NHES	National Health Examination Survey
NIDDM	Non-Insulin Dependent Diabetes Mellitus
NIH	National Institutes of Health
NTD	Neutral Tube Defect
OA	Osteoarthritis
PPA	Phenylpropanolamine
PT	Prothrombin Time
PTH	Parathyroid Hormone
RA	Rheumatoid Arthritis
RDA	Recommended Daily Allowance
RDI	Respiratory Disturbance Index
RMA	Resting Metabolic Rate
RMR	Resting Metabolic Rate
RNA	Ribonucleic Acid
RYGP-E	Roux-en-y gastric bypass
SQ	Subcutaneous
SSRI	Selective Seratonin Reuptake Inhibitor
TG	Triglyceride
TIBC	Total Iron Binding Capacity
TPN	Total Parenteal Nutrition
TSH	Thyroid Stimulating Hormone
UDP-N	UDP-N-Acetylglucosamine
UPPP	Uvulopalapharyngloplasty
USDA	US Department of Agriculture
UV	Ultraviolet
VBG	Vertical Banded Gastroplasty
WHR	Waist/Hip Ratio

INDEX